manual of RESPIRATORY CARE PROCEDURES

second edition

DIANE BLODGETT, C.R.T.I., R.R.T.

Formerly Technical Director, Respiratory Therapy, Faxton Hospital
Children's Hospital and Rehabilitation Center, Utica, New York

Acquisitions Editor: Lisa A. Biello
Sponsoring Editor: Delois Patterson
Manuscript Editor: Janet Greenwood
Indexer: Bernice Eisen
Design Director: Tracy Baldwin
Design Coordinator: Don Shenkle
Production Supervisor: J. Corey Gray
Production Coordinator: Charlene Catlett Squibb
Compositor: Bi-Comp, Incorporated
Printer/Binder: R. R. Donnelley & Sons Company

Second Edition

6   5   4   3   2   1

Library of Congress Cataloging-in-Publication Data

Blodgett, Diane.
    Manual of respiratory care procedures.

    Includes bibliographies and index.
    1. Respiratory therapy—Handbooks, manuals, etc.
I. Title. [DNLM: 1. Respiratory Therapy—handbooks.
WB 39 B652m]
RC735.I5B56   1987   616.2'004'636   86-21306
ISBN 0-397-50714-3

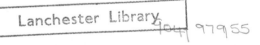
*The authors and publisher have exerted every effort to ensure that drug selec-
tion and dosage set forth in this text are in accord with current recommendations
and practice at the time of publication. However, in view of ongoing research,
changes in government regulations, and the constant flow of information relating to drug therapy and drug reactions, the reader is urged to check the package
insert for each drug for any change in indications and dosage and for added
warnings and precautions. This is particularly important when the recommended agent is a new or infrequently employed drug.*

To D.E.H.

contributors

Richard Branson, A.A.S., R.R.T.
Clinical Instructor
Department of Surgery
Division of Trauma/Critical Care
University of Cincinnati Hospitals
Cincinnati, Ohio

William DeForge, B.S., R.R.T., R.C.P.T.
Chief Technician
Cardiac Catheterization Laboratory
Norwalk Hospital
Norwalk, Connecticut

preface

Manual of Respiratory Care Procedures, Second Edition updates and refines the material presented in the first edition. The new illustrations and expanded appendix will further assist the student and practitioner in the day-to-day practice of respiratory care. All charts and tables have been revised. Because new information appears each month in our professional journals, I recommend that you WRITE IN THIS BOOK. Add to the guidelines. The contents are only guidelines that may someday become standards. Currently in respiratory care, we are seeing a thrust toward standardizing the care we give and the procedures we perform. I hope that by the next edition, more information about the scientific basis of respiratory care will be available so that procedures will be uniform. Until then, respiratory care practitioners are working toward refining and perfecting the profession—the goal for today and for the future.

Diane Blodgett, C.R.T.T., R.R.T.

preface to first edition

I undertook this project to provide the respiratory care practitioner with a guide to use at the bedside. Textbooks are left in the library, procedure manuals, in the technical director's office, and a helpful formula learned in a lecture, left on a pad somewhere in a locker. It was thus obvious to me that the practitioner needed a handbook that he could carry with him.

It is suggested, then, that the practitioner and student alike carry this procedure handbook with them—use it, write in it, revise it, and delete and add to it. I am not suggesting that all the information you need for your day-to-day respiratory care practice is here. I do, however, provide the reader with useful guidelines and procedures.

PLEASE WRITE IN THIS BOOK

It is for you, the respiratory practitioner.

There are areas that this book does not cover—primarily pediatrics—that must be addressed separately.

This guide should, however, provide most of the information needed in the clinical environment.

acknowledgments

To my contributors, Willie and Rich, who made this edition a lot easier.

To Lisa, thanks for being both an editor and a friend.

introduction to clinical respiratory care

Three essential components in the delivery of respiratory care are the patient, the procedure, and the outcome. Most of this book addresses the procedures. This introduction discusses the patient and the outcome of your procedures; but you, the practitioner, are directly involved in all three.

The Patient: Who is the patient? What is his medical problem, especially the problem that requires your intervention?

The Procedure: What did the physician have in mind when he ordered respiratory care? Did he make the appropriate choice? Will the chosen procedure help achieve the objectives of our care?

The Outcome: What should the outcome of our care be? How can we evaluate the outcome? How can we achieve our therapeutic objective in the most cost-effective way?

What you must know about your patient are the facts that will affect your interaction with him. Some facts will be immediately obvious when you enter the room: the patient is either male or female, old or young. Other data must be obtained from the chart: the diagnosis, history and physical, lab results, etc. Finally, more information can be obtained from the patient through dialogue and physical examination. Evaluate your patient before proceeding with any respiratory care.

All the information about the patient helps you to decide the therapeutic objectives. In each chapter, this book provides you with therapeutic objectives for each treatment modality. Knowing what each treatment regime can accomplish, you can match the care to the desired outcome. For example, if the patient has a history of left lower-lobe atelectasis, verified by physical finding and x-ray, then the objective is to reinflate that lung portion. How do you accomplish this task? The order should be written so that you achieve your goal for the patient. In this case, incentive spirometry followed by chest physiotherapy might be appropriate. Once the physician writes the order appropriate to the goal, then give the therapy following the standards of care for that treatment modality. At that time also identify the appropriate criteria for termination of the therapy. How will you know when to stop? When have the objectives been achieved? "Death or discharge" is never acceptable. An evaluation form, completed during the initial evaluation, helps the therapist to identify pertinent information needed about the respiratory care to be administered (see Evaluation Form on p. xviii).

To provide the best care to respiratory patients, the respiratory practitioner pays special attention when performing procedures. You must have a good grasp of the procedure, the benefits, any side-effects and hazards. You should explain the therapy to your patient to obtain full cooperation. As you administer the care, observe the patient for changes. Remember to use all your resources in order to maximize the benefits to the patient.

Once you know all about the patient and give the therapy, then you must evaluate the care you have given. Did the patient improve, remain unchanged, or get worse? How do you evaluate the patient?

PATIENT EVALUATION

Objective

To evaluate the respiratory care used to treat primary pulmonary disease or secondary pulmonary complications.

Procedure

Based on the specific problem that the patient has, use the following guidelines for evaluation.

Oxygenation: Evaluate oxygenation by checking vital signs and inspecting the lips, tongue, and extremities for signs of cyanosis. Since cyanosis is not obvious in all patients, sample arterial blood gases to evaluate oxygenation. You can also use oximetry or transcutaneous values once you have established a baseline. Oxygen therapy dosage can be titrated once you have the arterial blood gas sample result.

Ventilation: Auscultation gives you an easy method to quickly evaluate whether or not the patient is moving air throughout the lung fields. For those patients with primary lung disease, use simple spirometry (FVC, FEV_1) before and after therapy to indicate whether there is improvement. For those patients with respiratory insufficiency or failure, arterial blood gases are the most conclusive method of evaluating ventilation before and after the initiation of therapy ($PaCO_2$ = ventilation). Also, capnography or transcutaneous values can reflect ventilation.

Humidity and Aerosol Therapy: Evaluate sputum viscosity by comparing pre- and post-therapy sputum. Sputum color change can indicate improvement in the patient's ability to clear secretions. Auscultation can also indicate the effectiveness of therapy, especially when aerosolized medication has been administered for the relief of bronchospasm.

As the therapist, you must also know how to identify an adverse reaction.

GUIDELINES FOR IDENTIFYING AN ADVERSE REACTION DURING A RESPIRATORY CARE PROCEDURE

Objective

To identify an adverse reaction. Once you identify the adverse reaction, to take the appropriate action.

Procedure

The therapist should monitor changes in vital signs for change in pulse, change in blood pressure, change in respiration rate, and change in level of consciousness.

The therapist should monitor changes in physical signs for diaphoresis, cyanosis, increase in work of breathing, nausea or vomiting, vertigo, and decrease or change in breath sounds.

Once you identify an adverse reaction, look for the possible cause: bronchospasm, pneumothorax, cardiac arrest, bronchodilator overdose, improper teaching of the treatment, etc. Then take appropriate action.

For adverse changes in vital signs:

• Stop treatment.
• Report changes in vital signs to head nurse.
• Stay with patient until vital signs normalize.
• Chart adverse reaction and vital signs in patient's respiratory care record.

For adverse changes in physical signs:

• Stop treatment; stay with patient until stable.
• Inform head nurse.
• Administer oxygen for cyanosis or increased work of breathing.
• Maintain clear airway and initiate CPR if necessary.
• Chart adverse reaction in patient's respiratory care record.

If the adverse reaction is serious or life threatening, call for help and seek a physician's assistance immediately.

Finally, once you have come to know the patient, have given the therapy and evaluated the outcome, and have documented all aspects of the care provided, then communicate the information to other members of the health care team. Include in the respiratory care record the date and time therapy was given, the results of the care, and your signature. Include in the results of therapy vital signs (pre- and post-therapy breath sounds, notation about sputum or cough) and an overall evaluation of the therapy (oxygenation, ventilation, humidity and aerosol therapy). You also will want to note whether the patient was cooperative or not. If the patient refuses care or is unavailable, note in the record why the care was not provided. If the patient has an adverse reaction, document this along with the critical management. Also include in the record the results of any test you performed.

If you do all of these things—examine the patient, perform therapy according to accepted standards of respiratory care, evaluate the therapy results, and document what you do and the patient outcome—you meet the objective of your profession: to provide the patient with the optimum care. However, you are under another obligation in these days of federal regulations: you must provide the patient with the most appropriate care in the most cost-effective way. When you administer care that does not benefit the patient, you use time and resources that might be put to better use. Since you, the therapist or technician, are the best equipped to evaluate respiratory care, know the principles and standards and assist other health care providers in ordering and carrying out care that is cost effective and optimizes resources.

EVALUATION FORM
DEPARTMENT OF
RESPIRATORY CARE

Patient's Name _____ **Room #** _____

Age _____

Primary Diagnosis _____

Respiratory Diagnosis _____

Therapeutic Objectives of Respiratory Care:

_____

_____

_____

Respiratory Care Instructions Necessary to Achieve Objectives: (Type, Frequency, Duration, and Medication Order)

_____

_____

_____

_____

Criteria for Termination of Respiratory Care:

_____

_____

_____

Respiratory Care Record: (See Attached Forms)

Initiate Therapy:

    Signature: _____

    Date: _____

contents

manual of
respiratory care procedures

1

therapeutic gas administration
Diane Blodgett

The first section of this chapter deals with the delivery of therapeutic gases. The gases that are generally given by the respiratory therapist are oxygen and combinations of oxygen and carbon dioxide or oxygen and helium.

The therapeutic objectives for *oxygen* administration are to decrease myocardial work, decrease respiratory work, and relieve or prevent hypoxia. Hypoxia is the primary indication for the administration of oxygen. Administer oxygen when PaO_2 < 55, when there is evidence of cor pulmonale, when SaO_2 is less than 90% to 95%, or when the clinical record indicates hypoxemia. The etiology of hypoxia may involve an insufficient amount of oxygen crossing the alveolar capillary membrane (*hypoxic hypoxia*), an inability of blood to accept and transport sufficient oxygen (*hemic hypoxia*), a blood flow insufficient to provide oxygen to the tissues (*stagnant hypoxia*), an inability to utilize the oxygen at the tissue level (*histotoxic hypoxia*), and, finally, an inability to supply sufficient oxygen to meet the demand (*demand hypoxia*). The type and degree of hypoxia determine the appropriate device and concentration to use.

There are essentially no contraindications to the use of O_2; however, there are some hazards that accompany its use, especially when that use is excessive. These hazards include loss of hypoxic drive in the patient who chronically retains carbon dioxide and oxygen toxicity in patients who

1

TABLE 1-1. GAS ADMINISTRATION

GASES	INDICATIONS	DISEASE ENTITIES	GAS CONCENTRATIONS	DEVICES TO ADMINISTER GAS
Oxygen	1. Stagnant hypoxia	Shock Heart failure	35%–100%	Catheter, cannula, simple mask, partial rebreathing mask
	2. Histotoxic hypoxia	Cyanide poisoning	35%–100%, depending upon severity	Catheter, cannula, all masks
	3. Hemic hypoxia	Anemia Hemorrhage CO poisoning Methemoglobinemia	100%	Non-rebreathing mask
	4. Hypoxic hypoxia	High altitude Suffocation Drowning Pulmonary edema COPD	24%–100%	Catheter, cannula, all masks
	5. Demand hypoxia	Fever Exercise	24%–40%	Catheter, cannula, simple mask
Carbon dioxide/ oxygen	1. Low CO_2	Hiccups Hysteria	95% oxygen 5% carbon dioxide	Non-rebreathing mask
Helium/oxygen	1. Large airway obstruction	Tumor obstructing bronchus	70% helium/30% oxygen 80% helium/20% oxygen	Non-rebreathing mask
	2. Airway obstruction	COPD Asthma	80% helium/20% oxygen	Non-rebreathing mask

receive high levels of oxygen over a prolonged period of time (note that oxygen toxicity can occur in less than 24 hours). The CO_2 retainer appears lethargic, confused, somnolent, and has shallow respirations. ABGs reveal respiratory acidosis with or without hypoxemia. The patient with oxygen toxicity might complain of substernal pain, headache, cough, and even dyspnea. The physiological effects may include decreased ventilation as well as altered perfusion. Absorption atelectasis may appear. Generally, ABGs reveal a high PaO_2. There may be a decrease in vital capacity as well as arterial PO_2. Bronchopulmonary dysplasia and ARDS can occur, at times with inspired oxygen concentrations above 40; however, FIO_2 over 60 is more likely to cause problems. The criteria for termination of O_2 therapy include a stable cardiovascular system, acceptable blood gases on room air, and the elimination of the underlying disease causing hypoxia.

The therapeutic objectives for the administration of a mixture of *oxygen* and *carbon dioxide* are to restore CO_2 levels in hyperventilation hysteria and to treat hiccups. Mixtures of CO_2 (5%)/O_2 (95%) are usually administered intermittently (*i.e.,* QID) by non-rebreathing mask. The primary contraindication to O_2/CO_2 therapy is a patient's chronic CO_2 retention. The hazards include headache, depression, acute changes in vital signs (tachycardia, hypertension), and possible seizures and cardiac arrest. The criteria for the termination of therapy are the ability of the patient to control emotional status voluntarily and the cessation of hiccups.

The therapeutic objective for the administration of *oxygen* and *helium* is the relief of large or small airway obstruction. Mixtures of He (70%)/O_2 (30%) and He (80%)/O_2 (20%) are usually administered continuously by non-rebreathing mask. There are no contraindications to the administration of O_2/He mixtures. If high concentrations of oxygen are necessary, however, then the small concentration of He that might be added will be of little benefit. Concentrations of 70% to 80% helium are the most beneficial. Because helium is a safe, inert gas, there is only a minor problem with its administration—change in voice tone. The criterion for termination of therapy is the decrease in airway obstruction.

OXYGEN CATHETER

Description

An oxygen catheter is a smooth, flexible tube, approximately 16 inches in length. The catheter has multiple, well-spaced openings on the patient end.

Therapeutic Objective

To administer low to moderate concentrations of oxygen nasally.

Criteria for Termination

Stable cardiovascular system, acceptable ABGs on room air, elimination of the cause of hypoxia or hypoxemia.

Contraindication

None. See Hazards.

Procedure

1. Approach the patient and explain the procedure.
2. To determine the insertion depth of the catheter, mea-

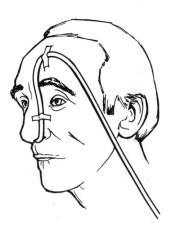

FIG. 1-1. *Oxygen catheter*

sure the distance from the patient's external nares to the end of the ear lobe.

3. With the humidifier, tubing, and catheter connected, set the oxygen flow at a low rate. (Humidifiers may be· unnecessary at low flows.)
4. Lubricate the catheter with a water-soluble lubricant. Check gas flow.
5. Determine the natural droop of the catheter.
6. With the oxygen still at low flow, insert the catheter along the floor of the nasal passage to the measured depth. Check placement by depressing tongue; if catheter is seen opposite uvula, pull back slightly (¼″).
7. Use adhesive strips to tape the catheter firmly to the side of the nose.
8. Adjust oxygen to desired flow.
9. Clip tubing to the bed sheet after allowing enough slack for the patient to move his head.
10. Evaluate effectiveness of oxygen by ABG, oximetry, or transcutaneous values.

Special Considerations

- Place "O_2/No Smoking" sign on entrance to patient's room.
- Encourage physician to obtain ABGs to monitor PaO_2.
- Do not permit smoking, sparks, flames, or ungrounded electrical equipment in area of oxygen use.

Hazards

- Nasal irritation
- Drying of the nasal mucosa
- Possible gastric distention
- Epistaxis

Flows and Inspired O_2 Concentrations

LITER FLOWS

One to six LPM yield O_2 concentrations of 22% to 50%, depending upon patient's ventilatory pattern.

Maintenance

• Every eight hours (at most) remove catheter and insert new one in alternate nostril, if possible.
• Discard catheter and tubing after use.

SMALL-BORE TUBING WITH CANNULA

Description

An over-the-ear nasal oxygen cannula is a bifurcated flexible tube that directs the oxygen flow into the nose by means of two plastic tips that fit into the nostrils.

Therapeutic Objective

To administer low to moderate oxygen concentrations nasally.

Criteria for Termination

Stable cardiovascular system, acceptable ABGs on room air, elimination of the cause of hypoxia or hypoxemia.

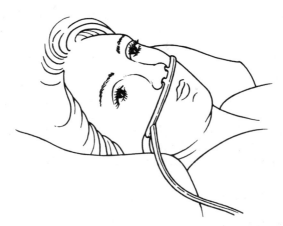

FIG. 1-2. *Nasal cannula (Bell CW, Blodgett D, Goike CA et al: Home Care and Rehabilitation in Respiratory Medicine, p 183. Philadelphia, JB Lippincott, 1984)*

Contraindications

Obstructed nasal passage; use mask. See Hazards.

Procedure

1. Approach the patient and explain the procedure.
2. With the humidifier, tubing, and cannula connected, set the oxygen flow at a low rate. (Humidifier may be unnecessary at low flows.)
3. Insert tips of cannula into nostrils.
4. Slip the two smaller plastic tubes over the ears and under the chin. Adjust the plastic slide until the cannula fits snugly and comfortably.
5. Clip tubing to clothes after allowing enough slack for patient to turn head.
6. Adjust oxygen flow to rate specified in physician's orders.
7. Evaluate effectiveness of oxygen by ABG, oximetry, or transcutaneous values.

Special Considerations

- Place "O_2/No Smoking" sign on entrance to patient's room.
- Encourage physician to obtain ABGs to monitor PaO_2 or monitor patient with oximeter or transcutaneous monitor.
- Nasal prongs may be cut shorter if uncomfortable for patient.
- This method of administration is effective only if the nasal passages are unobstructed. If one side is obstructed, expect lower FiO_2.
- Do not permit smoking, sparks, flames, or ungrounded electrical equipment in area of oxygen use.
- Check position of cannula prongs frequently.

Hazards

- Nasal irritation
- Drying of the nasal mucosa
- Sinus pain

- Epistaxis
- Cannula displacement

Flows and Inspired O_2 Concentrations

LITER FLOWS

One to six LPM yield O_2 concentrations of 22% to 50% depending upon patient's ventilatory pattern.

Maintenance

- Check the position of cannula tips frequently.
- Discard cannula and tubing after use.

SMALL-BORE TUBING AND SIMPLE MASK

Description

A simple mask is a flexible, cone-shaped device with a metal strip to mold the mask to the nose, an adjustable head strap, and multiple exhalation ports. The nasal mask covers the nasal openings.

Therapeutic Objective

To deliver medium concentrations of oxygen by mask.

Criteria for Termination

Stable cardiovascular system, acceptable ABGs on room air, elimination of the underlying cause of hypoxia or hypoxemia.

Contraindications

Patients who are at risk of vomiting; see Hazards.

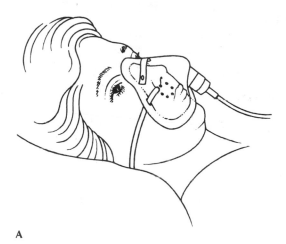

A

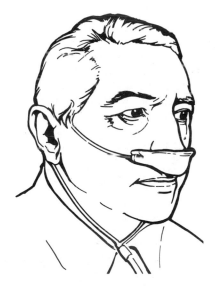

B

FIG. 1-3A: *Simple mask (Bell CW, Blodgett D, Goike CA et al: Home Care and Rehabilitation in Respiratory Medicine, p 183. Philadelphia, JB Lippincott, 1984);* **B:** *Nasal mask*

Procedure

1. Approach the patient and explain the procedure.
2. With the humidifier, tubing, and mask connected, set the oxygen at a low flow rate.
3. Place the mask on patient and carefully adjust headband so the fit is snug but not too tight.
4. Adjust the metal strip on the nose portion and mold mask to face (or position nasal mask).
5. Adjust O_2 flow to desired level. Minimum flow is 3 to 4 LPM (less flow with nasal mask).
6. Evaluate effectiveness of oxygen by ABG, oximetry, or transcutaneous values.

Special Considerations

- Place "O_2/No Smoking" sign on entrance to patient's room.
- Encourage physician to obtain ABGs to monitor PaO_2.
- Flow must be 3 to 4 LPM to eliminate CO_2.
- Do not permit smoking, sparks, flames, or ungrounded electrical equipment in area of oxygen use.

Hazards

- Aspiration with vomiting patient (except with nasal mask)
- Carbon dioxide accumulation at low-flow rate
- Subcutaneous emphysema into ocular tissue at high flow rate
- Pressure necrosis with tight-fitting masks
- Low FiO_2 if patient does not keep mask positioned correctly

Flows and Inspired O_2 Concentrations

LITER FLOWS

Three to ten LPM yield O_2 concentrations of 25% to 55% depending on minute ventilation and flow rate.

Maintenance

• Adjust mask PRN.
• Discard mask and tubing after use.

PARTIAL REBREATHING MASK WITH SMALL-BORE TUBING

Description

A partial rebreathing mask, a flexible, cone-shaped device with a reservoir bag attached, has an adjustable headstrap and a metal strip to mold the mask to the nose. The mask does not have one-way flap valves between bag and mask and on the exhalation ports (non-rebreathing mask has flap valves).

Therapeutic Objective

To administer medium to medium-high concentrations of oxygen by mask with reservoir bag.

Criteria for Termination

Stable cardiovascular system, acceptable ABGs on room air, elimination of hypoxia or hypoxemia.

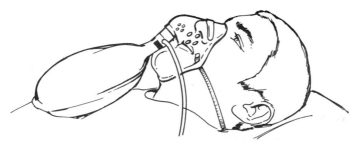

FIG. 1-4. *Partial rebreathing mask*

Contraindication

Patients who are at risk of vomiting; see Hazards.

Procedure

1. Approach the patient and explain the procedure.
2. With the humidifier, tubing, and mask connected, set the oxygen flow at a low rate.
3. Fill the reservoir bag with oxygen by occluding opening between bag and mask.
4. Slip mask on patient and slip strap around head.
5. Carefully adjust headband so that the fit is snug but not too tight.
6. Adjust the metal strip on the nose portion and mold mask to face.
7. Adjust oxygen flow so the bag will fill fully on exhalation and then almost collapse on inspiration.
8. Adjust flow to higher rate, if necessary, to maintain proper inflation of reservoir bag.
9. Evaluate effectiveness of oxygen by ABG, oximetry, or transcutaneous values.

Special Considerations

- Place "O_2/No Smoking" sign on entrance to patient's room.
- Encourage physician to obtain ABGs to monitor PaO_2.
- Do not permit smoking, sparks, flames, or ungrounded electrical equipment in area of oxygen use.
- If bag accumulates water, empty water from bag.
- Adjust mask as needed.

Hazards

- Aspiration with vomiting patient
- Pressure necrosis with tight-fitting mask
- Subcutaneous emphysema into ocular tissue at very high flows
- Carbon dioxide accumulation at low flows
- Low FIO_2 if patient does not keep mask in place

Flows and Inspired O_2 Concentrations

LITER FLOWS

Oxygen concentration of 35% to 75% can be achieved by adjusting flows to patient needs. The better the mask fit, the higher the concentration.

Maintenance

• If bag accumulates water, empty water out.
• Discard mask and tubing after use.

NON-REBREATHING MASK

Description

A non-rebreathing mask, a flexible, cone-shaped device with a reservoir bag attached, has a metal strip to mold the mask to the nose, an adjustable head strap, a flap valve between bag and mask, and flap valves on the exhalation ports.

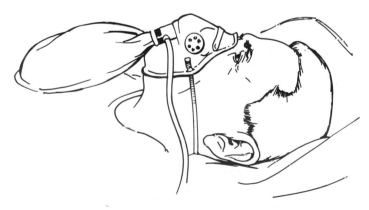

FIG. 1-5.　*Non-rebreathing mask*

Therapeutic Objective

To administer high concentrations of oxygen by mask with reservoir bag.

Criteria for Termination

Stable cardiovascular system, acceptable ABGs on room air, elimination of the underlying cause of hypoxia or hypoxemia.

Contraindications

Patients who are at risk of vomiting; see Hazards.

Procedure

1. Approach the patient and explain the procedure.
2. With the humidifier, tubing, and mask connected, set the oxygen flow at a low rate.
3. Fill the reservoir bag with oxygen by occluding the one-way valve between bag and mask.
4. Place mask on patient's face and slide head strap over head.
5. Carefully adjust headband so the fit is snug but not too tight.
6. Adjust the metal strip on the nose portion and mold mask to face.
7. Adjust oxygen flow so that the bag will fill on expiration and then almost collapse on inspiration.
8. Adjust flow to higher rate, if necessary, to ensure proper inflation of bag.
9. Evaluate effectiveness of oxygen by ABG, oximetry, or transcutaneous values.

Special Considerations

- Place "O_2/No Smoking" sign on entrance to patient's room.
- Encourage physician to obtain ABGs to monitor PaO_2.
- Make sure flap valves are not sticking.

• Do not permit smoking, sparks, flames, or ungrounded electrical equipment in area of oxygen use.

Hazards

• Aspiration with vomiting patient
• Subcutaneous emphysema into ocular tissue at very high flows
• Pressure necrosis with tight–fitting masks
• Suffocation due to insufficient flow
• Carbon dioxide accumulation at low flows
• Low FIO_2 if patient does not keep mask in place

Flows and Inspired O_2 Concentrations

The oxygen concentrations will be high; the better the mask fit, the higher the concentration

Concentrations of up to 95% can be achieved.

Flows must be sufficient to meet the patient's inspiratory demands.

Maintenance

• If bag accumulates water, empty water out.
• Discard mask and tubing after use.

SMALL-BORE TUBING WITH VENTURI MASK

Description

A venturi mask, a cone–shaped device with entrainment ports of various sizes at the base of the mask, has a metal strip to mold the mask to the nose, an adjustable head strap, and multiple exhalation ports.

Objective

To give a prescribed, precise low to medium concentration of oxygen by mask.

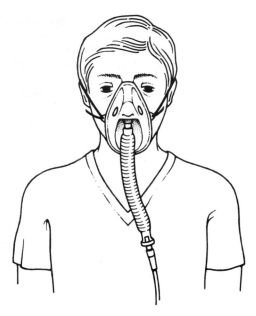

FIG. 1-6. *Venturi mask (Bell CW, Blodgett D, Goike CA et al: Home Care and Rehabilitation in Respiratory Care, p 184. Philadelphia, JB Lippincott, 1984)*

Criteria for Termination

Stable cardiovascular system, acceptable ABGs on room air, elimination of the underlying cause of hypoxia or hypoxemia.

Contraindications

Patients who are at risk of vomiting; see Hazards.

Procedure

1. Approach the patient and explain the procedure.
2. Attach tubing directly to flowmeter for low-concentra-

tion masks. Use humidifier for higher-concentration masks.
3. Adjust the flow of oxygen to that stated on the mask.
4. Place mask on patient's face and slide elastic strap over head.
5. Adjust the metal strip on the nose portion and mold mask to face.
6. Carefully adjust headband so the fit is snug but not too tight.
7. Evaluate effectiveness of oxygen by ABG, oximetry, or transcutaneous values.

Special Considerations

- Place "O_2/No Smoking" sign on entrance to patient's room.
- Encourage physician to obtain ABGs to monitor PaO_2.
- Be certain that venturi openings are always clear. Instruct the patient not to pull covers or sheets over the venturi openings.
- Do not permit smoking, sparks, flames, or ungrounded electrical equipment in area of oxygen use.

Hazards

- Aspiration with vomiting patient
- Pressure necrosis with tight-fitting mask
- Subcutaneous emphysema into ocular tissue at very high flows
- Low FiO_2 if patient is not wearing mask correctly

Flows and Inspired O_2 Concentrations

See Table 1-2.

Maintenance

- Maintain flow as indicated on mask.
- Discard mask and tubing after use.

TABLE 1-2.   FLOWS AND INSPIRED O$_2$ CONCENTRATIONS OF COMMON VENTURI MASKS

MASK %	LITER FLOW	AIR/O$_2$	TOTAL FLOW
24	4	20 : 1	84 LPM
28	4	10 : 1	44 LPM
31	6	7 : 1	49 LPM
35	8	5 : 1	48 LPM
40	8	3 : 1	32 LPM
50	12	1.75 : 1	33 LPM

AEROSOL MASK

Description

An aerosol mask, a flexible, cone-shaped device, has a metal strip to mold the mask to the nose, an adjustable head strap, two large openings for exhalation, and a large-bore tubing connection.

Therapeutic Objective

To administer, by mask, oxygen or air–oxygen mixtures saturated with water vapor at body temperature.

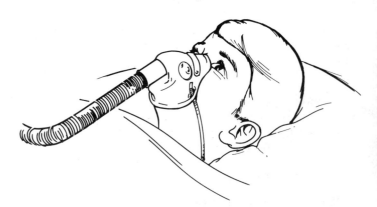

FIG. 1-7.   *Aerosol mask*

Criteria for Termination

When oxygen is used, same as oxygen. Zero humidity deficit, relief of inspiratory stridor. See Chapter 2: Aerosol and Humidity Therapy.

Contraindication

Patients who are at risk of vomiting; see Hazards.

Procedure

1. Approach patient and explain the procedure.
2. With the nebulizer or heated high humidifier, tubing, and mask connected, set the gas flow at 10 LPM.
3. Place mask on patient's face and slip strap around head.
4. Carefully adjust headband so that the fit is snug but not too tight.
5. Adjust the metal strip on the hose portion and mold mask to face.
6. Readjust flow to meet patient's needs. Mist should always be visible with aerosol.
7. Evaluate effectiveness of oxygen when FiO_2 is greater than 21%. Monitor ABG, oximetry, or transcutaneous values.

Special Considerations

- Make sure flow is adequate (mist visible with nebulizer).
- If oxygen is carrier gas, encourage physician to obtain ABGs to monitor PaO_2.
- If oxygen is carrier gas, place "O_2/No Smoking" sign on entrance to patient's room.
- Since output is high with nebulizer, make sure tubing is not blocked by water.
- Do not permit smoking, sparks, flames, or ungrounded electrical equipment in area of oxygen use.

Hazards

- Water accumulation in tubing
- Aspiration with vomiting patient

• Pressure necrosis with tight-fitting mask
• See hazards of high humidity and aerosol in Chapter 2.

Flows and Inspired O_2 Concentrations

Concentrations are stable when a venturi nebulizer is used at high flow rates. Concentrations delivered can be from 21% to 100%, depending on nebulizer settings and minute ventilation.

Maintenance

• Keep humidity or aerosol reservoir filled with sterile distilled water.
• Drain water from tubing when necessary. Do not drain back into reservoir.
• Wipe accumulated moisture from inside of mask when necessary.
• Discard tubing and mask after use.

FACE TENT

Description

The face tent, a shield-like device that fits under the chin and sweeps around the face, has an adjustable head strap and large-bore tubing connection.

Therapeutic Objective

To administer oxygen or air–oxygen mixtures saturated with water vapor at body temperature.

Criteria for Termination

When oxygen is used, same as oxygen. Zero humidity deficit, relief of inspiratory stridor. See Chapter 2: Aerosol and Humidity Therapy.

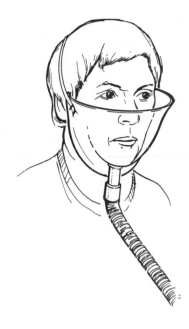

FIG. 1-8. *Face tent*

Contraindication

Patients who are at risk of vomiting; see Hazards.

Procedure

1. Approach the patient and explain the procedure.
2. With the nebulizer or heated high humidifier, tubing, and face tent connected, set the gas flow at 10 LPM (nebulizer setting determines FIO_2).
3. Slip strap around head and place tent under chin.
4. Carefully adjust headband so that the fit is snug but not too tight.
5. Readjust flow to meet patient's needs. Mist should always be visible with nebulizer.
6. When using supplemental O_2, evaluate effectiveness of oxygen by monitoring ABG, oximetry, or transcutaneous values.

Special Considerations

- Make sure flow is adequate (mist visible).
- If oxygen is carrier gas, encourage physician to obtain ABGs to monitor PaO_2. FiO_2 not predictable.
- If oxygen is carrier gas, place "O_2/No Smoking" sign on entrance to patient's room.
- Since output is high with nebulizer, make sure tubing is not blocked by water accumulation. Empty tubing when necessary; however, do not empty back into reservoir.
- Do not permit smoking, sparks, flames, or ungrounded electrical equipment in area of oxygen use.

Hazards

- Water accumulation in tubing blocking flow
- See humidity and aerosol therapy hazards in Chapter 2.

Flows and Inspired O_2 Concentrations

To stabilize concentrations, two nebulizers may be needed at high-flow rates. Concentrations delivered can be from 21% to 100% depending on nebulizer setting and gas source. FiO_2 impossible to predict.

Maintenance

- Keep jar filled with sterile distilled water or use prefilled nebulizer.
- When necessary, drain water from tubing.
- Discard tubing and face tent after use.

TRACH MASK

Description

A Trach mask is a flexible, collar-shaped device with an adjustable neck strap, large-bore tubing connection, and large exhalation port.

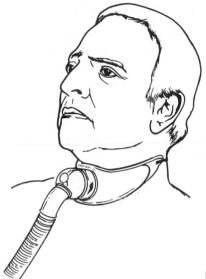

FIG. 1-9. *Trach mask*

Therapeutic Objective

To deliver oxygen or air–oxygen mixtures saturated with water vapor at body temperature to the patient with a tracheostomy or laryngectomy.

Criteria for Termination

When oxygen is used, same as oxygen. Zero humidity deficit. See Chapter 2: Humidity and Aerosol Therapy.

Contraindication

None. See Hazards.

Procedure

1. Approach the patient and explain the procedure.
2. With the nebulizer or heated high humidifier, tubing,

and trach mask attached, set the gas flow at 10 LPM (nebulizer setting will determine FiO_2).
3. Slip strap around patient's neck.
4. Adjust strap so mask lies loosely in front to meet patient's needs.
5. Readjust flow to meet patient's needs.
6. When using supplemental O_2, evaluate effectiveness of oxygen by monitoring ABG, oximetry, or transcutaneous values.

Special Considerations

• Make sure flow is adequate (mist visible).
• If oxygen is carrier gas, encourage physician to obtain ABGs to monitor PaO_2.
• If oxygen is carrier gas, place "O_2/No Smoking" sign on entrance to patient's room.
• Monitor temperature when using high humidity or aerosol therapy.
• Since output is high with nebulizer, make sure tubing is not blocked by water accumulation. Empty tubing when necessary but not back into reservoir.
• Do not permit smoking, sparks, flames, or ungrounded electrical equipment in area of oxygen use.

Hazards

• Water accumulation in tubing
• Infection
• Pulmonary or tracheal burns when aerosol or high humidity is heated
• Local irritation
• See hazards of high humidity and aerosol therapy in Chapter 2.

Flows and Inspired O_2 Concentrations

Concentrations are fairly stable when a venturi nebulizer or high humidifier is used at high flow rates. Concentrations delivered can be from 21% to 100% depending on nebulizer setting and gas source. High humidifiers can use any primary or blended source gas.

Maintenance

- Keep jar filled with sterile distilled water.
- Drain water when necessary; do not drain back into reservoir.
- Discard tubing and trach mask after use.

AEROSOL T-TUBE

Description

Plastic T-adapter with 15-mm connection that fits directly to tracheostomy or endotracheal tube. Large-bore tubing transmits the aerosol or high humidity to the T-tube.

Therapeutic Objective

To administer oxygen or air–oxygen mixtures saturated with water vapor at body temperature.

Criteria for Termination

When oxygen is used, same as oxygen. Zero humidity deficit. See Chapter 2: Aerosol and Humidity Therapy.

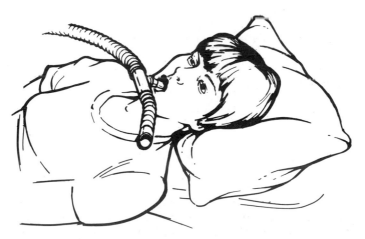

FIG. 1-10. *Aerosol T-adapter*

Contraindications

None. See Hazards.

Procedure

1. Approach the patient and explain the procedure.
2. With the nebulizer or heated high humidifier, tubing, and T-tube connected, set the gas flow at 10 LPM (nebulizer setting will determine FiO_2).
3. Attach the T-tube to the endotracheal tube or tracheostomy tube.
4. Readjust flow to meet patient's needs. Mist should always be visible.
5. Evaluate the effectiveness of oxygen when FiO_2 is greater than 21%. Monitor ABG, oximetry, or transcutaneous values.

Special Considerations

- Add reservoir tube on exhalation side of T-tube to maintain stable oxygen concentration.
- Make sure flow is adequate (mist visible with nebulizer).
- Heating the mist is advisable.
- If oxygen is carrier gas, encourage physician to obtain ABGs to monitor PaO_2.
- If oxygen is carrier gas, place "O_2/No Smoking" sign on entrance to patient's room.
- Since output is high with nebulizer or high humidifier, make sure tubing is not blocked by water accumulation. Do not empty accumulated water back into reservoir.
- Do not permit smoking, sparks, flames, or ungrounded electrical equipment in area of oxygen use.

Hazards

- Water accumulation in tubing
- Overhydration
- Pulmonary or tracheal burns when reservoir is heated
- Blockage of T-tube with secretions
- Infection

Flows and Inspired O_2 Concentrations

Concentrations are stable when a venturi nebulizer is used at high flow rates. Concentrations delivered can be from 24% to 100% depending upon nebulizer setting and source gas. High humidifiers can use any primary or blended gas source.

Maintenance

• Keep jar filled with sterile distilled water.
• Drain water when necessary.
• Discard tubing and T-tube after use.

AEROSOL TENT (CROUPETTE)

Description

The aerosol tent, an enclosure device, consists of a plastic canopy, a cooling or circulating unit, and a nebulizer.

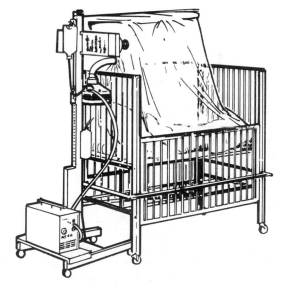

FIG. 1-11. *Aerosol tent*

Therapeutic Objective

To provide a high-humidity environment, with or without oxygen enrichment, cooled to 6 to 15 degrees below ambient. The primary application is for infants or youths who will not accept other gas administration devices.

Criteria for Termination

Zero humidity deficit; same as oxygen when oxygen is used. See Chapter 2: Humidity and Aerosol Therapy.

Contraindications

Patients who need stable oxygen atmosphere while requiring significant nursing care; patients who will not tolerate confined space.

Procedure

1. Approach the patient and explain the procedure.
2. Position cooling nebulizer unit on crib or bed.
3. Attach canopy to unit and position over bed.
4. Fill ice chamber or start refrigeration unit.
5. Fill nebulizer reservoir with sterile distilled water.
6. Set flow through nebulizer to at least 10 LPM (source gas and nebulizer dilution will determine FIO_2). Run unit for 5 to 10 minutes to flush system.
7. Place patient in tent.
8. Tuck in canopy sides under mattress. Fold sheet over front portion of the tent edge.
9. Adjust flow when patient has settled.

Special Considerations

- Make sure gas flow is sufficient.
- Keep canopy tucked in and closed to maintain stable environment.
- If oxygen is used as carrier gas, monitor FIO_2, either continuously or q4h.

- If oxygen is carrier gas, encourage physician to obtain ABGs or use oximetry or transcutaneous values.
- If oxygen is carrier gas, place "O_2/No Smoking" sign on entrance to patient's room.
- Do not permit smoking, sparks, flames, or ungrounded electrical equipment in area of oxygen use.
- Do not permit friction toys in tent.
- Canopy can be closed- or open-topped. Cut hole in roof of canopy to allow heat to rise.

Hazards

- Carbon dioxide accumulation at low flow.
- Unstable oxygen concentrations when enclosure is opened.
- Fire with supplementary oxygen.
- With high humidity atmosphere (using high-output nebulizer), fluid overload and loss of patient visibility are possible hazards.
- Infection.

Flows and Inspired O_2 Concentrations

Concentrations of 21% to 60% are obtainable, depending on flow rate, tightness of enclosure, and venturi setting.

Maintenance

- Keep nebulizer jar filled with sterile distilled water.
- Ice chamber must be kept filled with a combination of ice and water. Do not drain chamber until last cube has melted; then replace with combination of water and ice.
- Bedding and patient clothes may need frequent changing as a result of dampness.

□ PRIMARY GAS SOURCE DEVICES

This section deals with the equipment that supplies the therapeutic gases. Tanks, compressors, piping systems, concentrators, blenders, and the equipment that controls the pressure and flow of gas are all covered in the following procedures.

The previous section of this chapter presented the therapeutic uses of various gases, gas mixtures, and the devices necessary to administer the gases. Now we need to know how to use and control the sources of the gas that we use. In some instances, a less complex piece of equipment, such as a compressor or concentrator, supplies the gas. The more complicated system may require two gas sources and a blender to deliver a precise mixture of air and oxygen.

Whatever the source gas, this section will review the procedures for its use and the necessary safety standards that must be followed.

TANKS/CYLINDERS

Description

Cylinders and tanks for storage of medical gases are available in sizes from AA to H or K. These gas sources supply medical gases in a portable container to the patient. The tanks are generally color-coded, have markings that identify their contents, and have standardized valve outlet fittings (see Tables 1-3, 1-4, 1-5, and 1-6).

TABLE 1-3. COLOR CODING FOR CYLINDERS

Oxygen (O_2)—Green

Carbon dioxide (CO_2)—Gray

Carbon dioxide/Oxygen (CO_2/O_2)—Gray/Green

Nitrous oxide (N_2O)—Blue

Helium (He)—Brown

Helium/Oxygen (He/O_2)—Brown/Green

Cyclopropane (C_3H_6)—Orange

Ethylene (C_2H_4)—Red

Nitrogen (N_2)—Black

Nitrogen/Oxygen (N_2/O_2)—Black/Orange

TABLE 1-4. GAS CATEGORIES

Oxygen—Oxidant
Carbon dioxide—Inert
Cyclopropane—Flammable
Ethylene–Ethylene oxide—Flammable
Helium—Inert
Nitrogen—Inert
Nitrous oxide—Oxidant

TABLE 1-5. PIN INDEX SAFETY SYSTEM COMBINATIONS

GAS	PIN CONFIGURATIONS
Oxygen	2–5
Carbon dioxide/Oxygen (less than 7%)	2–6
Carbon dioxide/Oxygen (more than 7%)	1–6
Nitrous oxide	3–5
Helium/Oxygen (less than 80%)	2–4
Helium/Oxygen (more than 80%)	4–6
Cyclopropane	3–6
Ethylene	1–3
Air, medical	1–5

TABLE 1-6. DIAMETER INDEX SAFETY SYSTEM NUMBERS

GAS	CONNECTIONS
Oxygen	1240
Carbon dioxide	1080
Carbon dioxide/Oxygen (less than 7%)	1080
Carbon dioxide/Oxygen (more than 7%)	1200
Nitrous oxide	1040
Helium	1060
Helium/Oxygen (less than 20%)	1060
Helium/Oxygen (more than 20%)	1180
Cyclopropane	1100
Ethylene	1140
Air, medical	1160
Suction	1220

Objective

To provide medical gases in a portable unit.

Procedure

The following procedures are used in conjunction with medical gas cylinders.

GENERAL STORAGE PROCEDURES

1. Follow all National Fire Prevention Association regulations for storage. Local regulations and codes may further restrict storage of gases.

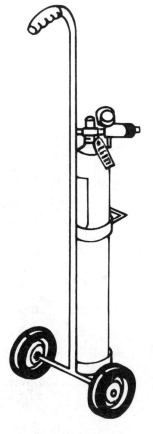

FIG. 1-12. *E-cylinder on cart (Bell CW, Blodgett D, Goike CA et al: Home Care and Rehabilitation in Respiratory Medicine, p 187. Philadelphia, JB Lippincott, 1984)*

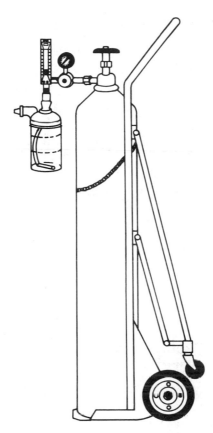

FIG. 1-13. *K-cyclinder on cart (Bell CW, Blodgett D, Goike CA et al· Home Care and Rehabilitation in Respiratory Medicine, p. 181. Philadelphia, JB Lippincott, 1984)*

2. Separate flammable gases from all other gases (store in separate areas).
3. Store full and empty cylinders separately.
4. Store oxygen and nitrous oxide in a well-vented (to the outside), cool, dry, and fire-resistant area.
5. Make provisions so that tanks cannot be knocked over.
   a. Chain larger cylinders to wall.
   b. Provide racks for smaller cylinders.

6. Do not store cylinders in the operating room.
7. Store cylinders so they are protected from extreme weather conditions.
8. Keep caps in place during storage.

TRANSPORTATION: IN-HOSPITAL GUIDELINES

1. Transport tanks on carts provided for that use.
2. Transport tanks in the upright position.
3. Secure the tank on the cart with chain or strap.
4. Push the cart so that you have maximum handling abilities (do not pull).

USAGE: IN-HOSPITAL GUIDELINES

1. Always crack cylinders to remove lint or soil from the cylinder outlet. Crack tank away from you.
2. Turn tanks on slowly to dissipate heat. Open valve fully and back ¼ turn.
3. Never allow oil, grease, or fuel of any type to come in contact with cylinder valves or regulators.
4. Post "No Smoking" signs on tanks and directly outside the room where oxygen is in use. Do not permit open flames, sparks, or smoking in this area.
5. When using oxygen with a controlled-environment device, do not use electrical or battery-operated equipment or toys (*i.e.,* call bells, TV control, friction toys).
6. Test for system leaks with solution of soapy water. Watch for bubbles.

Special Considerations

• Read label to identify gas.
• Do not use if label cannot be read or has been removed.
• Do not depend on color-coding for identification.

$$\text{E-cylinder duration of flow} = \frac{0.28 \times \text{gauge pressure}}{\text{liters per minute gas flow}}$$

$$\text{H- or K-cylinder duration of flow} = \frac{3.14 \times \text{gauge pressure}}{\text{liters per minute gas flow}}$$

Hazards

• Fire
• Explosion

- Personal injuries due to incorrect handling of cylinders
- Administration of inappropriate gas if tank is not clearly identified by labeling

Maintenance

- Isolate and return to supplier any tanks that appear damaged.
- Keep tanks in approved storage areas and set aside for that use only. Keep storage area clean with signs in full view.
- Follow all regulations regarding the safe use and handling of gases.
- Never attempt to repair cylinder valves or safety relief devices.
- Replace cylinders when contents read below 500 PSIG.
- Wipe tanks to remove dust and dirt before placing in use.

REDUCING VALVES: FLOWMETERS/REGULATORS

Description

A full cylinder of a medical gas may have a pressure of more than 2000 PSIG. Before the gas from the cylinder can be used safely, a pressure-reducing regulator must be attached to the cylinder. The reducing valve reduces the high pressure from a cylinder in one, two, or three stages. The flowmeter, which can be attached to the reducing valve, is calibrated to indicate liter flow. A flowmeter can be compensated, uncompensated, or a Bourdon gauge. A regulator is a reducing valve and flowmeter in combination.

Objective

To reduce the high pressures in a cylinder to working pressures and to control the rate of flow of a gas to the patient.

Procedure

The following procedures are used in conjunction with reducing valves, regulators, and flowmeters.

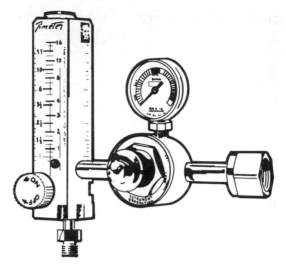

FIG. 1-14. *Regulator (large tank)*

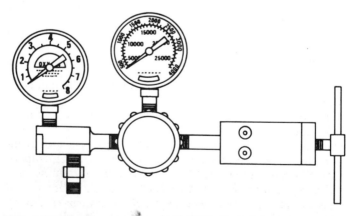

FIG. 1-15. *Regulator (small tank) (Bell CW, Blodgett D, Goike AC et al: Home Care and Rehabilitation in Respiratory Medicine, p 187. Philadelphia, JB Lippincott, 1984)*

ATTACHMENT OF REGULATOR

1. Identify the cylinder by reading the label.
2. Obtain the appropriate regulator for the gas.
3. Crack cylinder to remove dust or lint from valve opening. (Small cylinders: Remove cover seal from pin index configuration.)
4. Attach regulator to cylinder connection and tighten the nut firmly by hand. Tighten slightly with wrench if necessary. (Small cylinders: Place yoke of regulator over cylinder valve. Set pins of regulator into pin holes on cylinder. Tighten wing bolt.)

TURNING ON REGULATOR

1. Open cylinder valve slowly.
2. Read contents of tank. Replace if below 500 PSIG. Label empty tanks.
3. Connect oxygen–administrating device to flowmeter outlet.
4. Turn on flowmeter to prescribed flow rate. Read flow rate at center of ball.

TURNING OFF REGULATOR

1. Close cylinder valve slowly.
2. When flow reads zero, turn adjustment on flowmeter to the off position.

Special Considerations

- Do not use oil or grease for lubrication of regulators or flowmeters.
- Do not interchange regulators from one gas to another.
- Do not use adaptors.
- Gauges on regulators are Bourdon gauges, indicating pressure. Thorpe tubes on regulators are either compensated or uncompensated flowmeters and indicate flows.
- Use regulators with compensated Thorpe tubes for all gas–delivering situations except patient transport; during patient transport a regulator with a Bourdon gauge should be used. Bourdon gauges can be read in any position.

- Read flowmeter (pressure–compensated) on middle of indicator ball.
- Flowmeters are usually calibrated from 0 to 7 LPM or 0 to 15 LPM.
- Flowmeters can be used directly with piped systems.
- Flowmeters may incorporate high-pressure outlet.
- Never use oil on oxygen valve, regulator, or with any equipment using oxygen.

Hazards

- Fire
- Explosion
- Inaccurate flow rates with uncompensated flowmeter or Bourdon gauge when there is back pressure

Maintenance

- Do not use equipment that shows signs of damage or wear.
- Equipment should be repaired only by trained personnel.
- Store equipment in dust-free area.

PIPED-GAS SOURCES: WALL OUTLETS

Description

The bulk gas system supplies a medical gas to the patient at the bedside. The gases that are generally provided at the bedside are oxygen, air, and vacuum. Nitrogen and nitrous oxide may also be piped into the operating room. The wall outlets should provide keyed connections so that incorrect gas administration cannot be inadvertently given. Flowmeters are used to regulate gas flow from the wall to the patient. High-pressure lines provide gas source to mechanical devices such as IPPB and CMV apparatus.

Objective

To provide a compact, efficient method of administering therapeutic gases at the bedside.

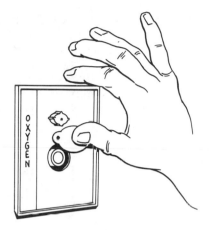

FIG. 1-16. *Wall outlet: DISS*

Procedure

CONNECTION OF EQUIPMENT TO DIAMETER INDEX SAFETY SYSTEM (DISS) OUTLETS

1. Turn equipment (flowmeter/vacuum) to the off position.
2. Fasten equipment to wall outlet by twisting the female DISS adapter clockwise onto the wall male DISS adapter.
3. Turn on equipment. Adjust flowmeter or vacuum setting to appropriate position.

DISCONNECTION OF EQUIPMENT FROM DISS OUTLETS

1. Turn equipment to the off position.
2. When the indicator has dropped back to zero, unfasten the female DISS adapter from the wall male adapter by turning counterclockwise.
3. If possible, replace dust cap on wall outlet.

CONNECTION OF EQUIPMENT TO QUICK-CONNECT OUTLETS

1. Close the flow–adjusting valve of the flowmeter or vacuum regulator.

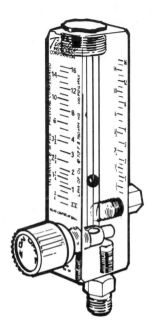

FIG. 1-17.   *Flowmeter*

2. Insert the wall inlet of the flowmeter into the opening of the outlet and make a firm connection.
3. Slowly open the flow-adjusting valve of the flowmeter (adjust vacuum regulator). As the oxygen flows into the flowmeter, the float will rise. Read flow at center of ball.

DISCONNECTION OF EQUIPMENT FROM QUICK-CONNECT OUTLETS

1. Turn equipment to the off position.
2. Release equipment from wall valve socket. Some releases are initiated by pushing a button on wall, others by pulling retainer housing back or by pressing a release button on the housing.
3. If possible, replace dust cap on wall outlet.

Special Considerations

• Some flowmeters have a high-pressure outlet incorporated in them.
• Quick-connect adapters are available in Diamond, Schra-

der, NCG, Puritan, OES, and Hansen configurations.
Each differs slightly from the others.
- Post "No Smoking/Oxygen in Use" signs on door and at patient's bedside.
- Compressed air outlets may require water trap to collect condensation.
- Use air flowmeter with air. Use oxygen flowmeter with oxygen.

Hazards

- Contaminated piped gases
- Low or high pressures in piping system

Maintenance

- Report leaks in wall outlets to appropriate personnel.
- Check wall outlets periodically to make certain that line pressures are being maintained at each outlet.
- Whenever piped outlets have been changed or added, analyze gas and check line pressure.

AIR COMPRESSORS

Description

Air compressors are devices used to provide a source of air. They are of three types: piston, diaphragm, and rotary. The compressors may provide an external or internal source of air for respiratory therapy equipment.

Objective

To provide a source of medical air to power respiratory therapy equipment.

Procedure

Most of these devices have an on and off switch with a control knob to adjust pressure or flow.

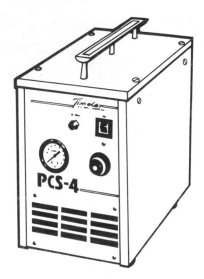

FIG. 1-18. *Compressor*

1. Connect compressor power line to electrical outlet.
2. Connect gas–administering equipment to outlet of compressor.
3. Turn on compressor.
4. Adjust flow or pressure to meet the needs of the equipment and patient.

Special Considerations

• Choose the appropriate compressor to meet the needs of the equipment to be powered. Not all compressors will be able to power a respirator, large-volume nebulizer, or blender.
• Most compressors have oxygen DISS outlets for connection to gas–administration devices.

Hazards

• Overheating
• Provision of air to patients requiring oxygen
• Insufficient pressure or flow for needs of respiratory therapy device or patient's needs

Maintenance

• Refer to service manual if compressor cannot reach desired pressure, is noisy, or overheats.
• Empty water or condensation trap PRN.
• Clean inlet filters daily.

OXYGEN BLENDER

Description

An oxygen blender controls precise oxygen concentrations to within 3% of indicated setting. This device is operated with the use of a 50 PSI air and 50 PSI oxygen inlet gas pressure source. The blender is a high-flow source of gas. (Some models have low-flow modules or connections.)

Objective

To deliver a precise concentration of an air–oxygen mixture through respiratory therapy equipment.

Procedure

1. Mount blender to ventilator, wall, or other stable structure.

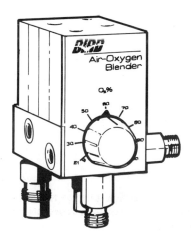

FIG. 1-19. *Blender*

2. Connect inlet pressure hoses to blender according to the DISS connections for air and oxygen.
3. Connect each inlet hose to its separate 50 PSI gas source (wall outlet or tank for oxygen and wall outlet, tank or compressor for compressed air).
4. Connect equipment to outlet fitting.
5. Turn on both 50 PSI gas sources.
6. Regulate air–oxygen concentration with front dial to desired percentage.
7. Monitor FiO_2 to verify setting.

Special Considerations

- Low-flow module must be provided or special adjustments must be made on blenders to be used for gas flows less than 15 LPM.
- Many blenders have alarm systems to indicate when one source gas is low.
- Use water trap for air sources.
- DISS standard fittings for air and oxygen on all blenders.

Hazards

- Failure of one gas source can allow use of the higher pressure gas source as the means of providing flow to the patient.
- Not all blenders may be able to meet peak or high demands. FiO_2 may fluctuate with high demand.

Maintenance

- Inlet filters should be checked periodically.
- Check oxygen concentrations with settings on blender to verify controls.

OXYGEN CONCENTRATOR

Description

This device extracts oxygen from room air and provides the patient with a continuous flow of oxygen-enriched air.

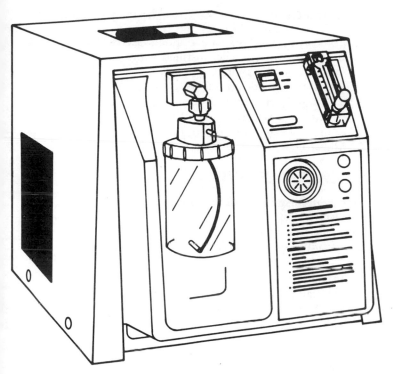

FIG. 1-20. *Oxygen concentrator (Bell CW, Blodgett D, Goike AC et al: Home Care and Rehabilitation in Respiratory Medicine, p 193. Philadelphia, JB Lippincott, 1984)*

Therapeutic Objective

To provide the patient with a source of oxygen-enriched air. To limit the use of cylinders for the home oxygen therapy patient.

Criteria for Termination

Same as oxygen.

Contraindication

When patient needs high FIO_2.

Procedure

1. Connect power line to grounded electrical source. Fill humidifier with sterile, distilled water.
2. Turn on power switch.
3. Adjust flow to desired level.
4. Check oxygen concentration on analyzer. Adjust the flowmeter if necessary.
5. Connect oxygen-administrating device to patient.
6. Adjust flow rate; see manufacturer's guidelines.

Special Considerations

- Generally used for home use for those patients who need low-flow oxygen.
- May be noisy for the light sleeper.
- Most units available with oxygen analyzer.
- Use humidifiers to prevent nasal mucosa irritation when flows are greater than 1.5 LPM.
- Small cylinder backup should always be available.
- Alarms indicate low oxygen output or power failure.
- OECO system provides high humidity, high flow rates with low FiO_2s.

Hazards

- Electrical line failure
- Inadequate oxygen supply for patients who need high concentrations of oxygen at high flow rates

Maintenance

- Oxygen analyzer fuel cell needs periodic replacement.
- Clean lint and dust filters PRN.
- Keep humidifier clean and filled with sterile, distilled water when in use. Clean daily.
- Use electrical line failure alarm in line.

BIBLIOGRAPHY

Brown M, Ziment I: Evaluation of an oxygen concentration in patients with COPD. Respir Ther 8, No. 5: 55, 1978

Burton GG, Hodgkin JG: Respiratory Care: A Guide to Clinical Practice. Philadelphia, JB Lippincott, 1984

Fisher A: Oxygen therapy side effects and toxicity. Am Rev Respir Dis (Suppl) 122, No. 5: 61–69, 1980

Fluck R: Letter: Causes of CO_2 retention in COPD patients breathing supplemental oxygen. Resp Care 29: 167, 1984

Hess D et al: Effect of nasal cannula displacement on arterial oxygen tension. Resp Care 29, No. 1: 21–24, 1984

Luce JM: Long term oxygen therapy: Physiologic and economic considerations. Resp Care 28, No. 7: 866–875, 1983

Mathewson H: Carbon dioxide: Therapeutic for what? Resp Care 27, No. 10: 1272, 1982

Mathewson H: Helium: Who needs it? Resp Care 27, No. 11: 1400–1401, 1982

Mathewson H: Pulmonary oxygen toxicity: Potential and protectors. Resp Care 29, No. 7: 760–762, 1984

Monast R, Kaye W: Problems in delivering desired oxygen concentrations from jet nebulizers to patients via face tents. Resp Care 29, No. 10: 994–1000, 1984

Tierney D: Oxygen therapy: Summary. Am Rev Respir Dis (Suppl) 122, No. 5: 15–16, 1980

Trep B, Nicotra B, Carter R, Phillips R, Otsap B: Evaluation of an oxygen conserving nasal cannula. Resp Care 30, No. 1: 19–25, 1985

Ward J, Gracey D: Arterial oxygen values achieved by COPD patients breathing oxygen alternately via nasal mask and nasal cannula. Resp Care 30, No. 4: 250–255, 1985

Whipple T, and Lusk R: A device for administering low flow oxygen to patients with tracheostomies. Resp Care 30, No. 4: 266–267, 1985

2

aerosol and humidity therapy

Diane Blodgett

Most respiratory care modalities incorporate a humidifying or an aerosol-generating device. There are exceptions (*e.g.,* chest physiotherapy), but even these treatments may be preceded by aerosol or high-humidity therapy.

The basic difference between humidifiers and aerosol generators is that humidifying units increase the water vapor content (molecular water) while aerosol generators create liquid suspended in a gas (particulate water).

The therapeutic objectives of humidity therapy are to humidify inspired gases and to prevent the loss of water vapor from the respiratory tract. The criteria for termination of humidity therapy are discontinuation of the inspiration of dry gases and the ability of the patient to maintain a neutral or slightly positive water balance.

The objectives of aerosol therapy differ because while humidity therapy prevents respiratory water loss, aerosol therapy adds water to the respiratory system. The therapeutic objectives of aerosol therapy include humidifying inspired gases, hydrating the respiratory system, aiding in the liquification of retained dry secretions, inducing a cough to obtain a sputum specimen or promote bronchial hygiene, providing a method of delivering medication into the tracheobronchial tree, and decreasing laryngeal edema.

The criteria for termination of aerosol therapy are a normal fluid balance (0 humidity deficit), use of the normal anatomical humidification system (extubation), normal auscultatory sounds, ability to mobilize secretions independently, relief of bronchospasm, and relief of inspiratory stridor.

TABLE 2-1a. THERAPEUTIC OBJECTIVES
Therapeutic Objectives for Humidity Therapy
Humidify inspired gases
Prevent loss of water vapor from the respiratory tract
Therapeutic Objectives for Aerosol Therapy
Deliver medication into the tracheobronchial tree
Decrease laryngeal edema
Induce a cough to obtain a specimen
Hydrate the respiratory system

Each type of therapy may be given heated or unheated, either intermittently or continuously. Humidifiers are usually utilized on a continuous basis for gas administration and for mechanical ventilation. The advantages of humidifiers are that there is little chance of bacterial contamination and that the devices are simple to use and maintain. The disadvantage is the low relative humidity provided unless the unit is heated. Standard unheated bubble humidifiers are cool (less than 26°C) and dry (less than 30% relative humidity at body temperature). Simple nonheated humidifiers may provide close to 100% relative humidity at their operating temperature, which may be in the 17°–20°C range; however, this amount of moisture supplies only about one third of the total moisture needed for the respiratory tract's humidification at body temperature.[1] Humidifiers in the bubble classification are most efficient at low flow rates (2.5–5.0 LPM). At these flow rates the bubblers may be expected to deliver between 38% to 48% relative humidity at body temperature; the output from bubble humidifiers is small (14.6–20.4 mg/l).[2] Whether the molecular water contribution of unheated bubble humidifiers can correct a humidity deficit is debatable, but it is generally agreed that, in contrast to dry gas therapy, it can prevent a humidity deficit from worsening.[3] Tanks, bulk systems, concentrators, and liquid systems, all start with a relative humidity at the outflow of zero or near zero.

Aerosol generators are used on an intermittent basis to meet the previously mentioned therapeutic objectives, except for hydration of the respiratory system. In this in-

TABLE 2-1b. COMPARISON OF AEROSOL AND HUMIDITY THERAPY

THERAPY	OBJECTIVE	CRITERIA FOR TERMINATION
Aerosol therapy (intermittent)	Deposit pharmacologic agent in upper or lower airway	Relief of bronchospasm
	Thin secretions	Clearing of adventitious breath sounds
	Induce a productive cough	Ability to raise own secretions
Humidity therapy	Humidify inspired gases	Zero humidity deficit
	Decrease humidity deficit	Discontinuation of therapeutic gas administration (simple or ventilator)
	Prevent loss of water vapor from respiratory tract	
Aerosol therapy (continuous)	Decrease laryngeal edema	Relief of inspiratory stridor
	Decrease humidity deficit	Normal fluid balance
		Extubation: (use of normal anatomical humidification system)
	Thin secretions	Normal fluid balance

stance, continuous aerosol may be appropriate, although heated humidifiers are the equipment of choice. Do not use aerosols when humidification is the only goal since microorganisms may be provided a carrier by the particulate matter to transport them into the respiratory tract. Do use aerosols when liquid volume or medication deposition is required. Aerosol generators deposit a large amount of solution into both the upper and lower airways and deliver medications to be administered topically, thereby meeting the therapeutic objectives. There are some disadvantages to aerosol units. The aerosol can produce a reflex bronchospasm, can become a vehicle for bacteria transmission, and in some instances, can provide too much liquid for the cardiorespiratory system (overhydration). Additionally, bland aerosols have not been shown to accomplish any therapeutic task.[4] Whatever the device chosen, the therapist should weigh the advantages and disadvantages of each method of therapy and choose the treatment modality which best accomplishes the goal while providing the optimum level of patient care and safety. Evaluation of the patient following the administration of therapy will help the therapist judge the appropriateness of the treatment.

HEATERS FOR HUMIDIFIERS AND AEROSOL GENERATORS

Description

Aerosol or humidifier heaters raise the temperature of the liquid in the reservoir. As the temperature of the liquid increases, the relative humidity and output increase.

Objectives

To increase the relative humidity to 100% at body temperature. To increase the nebulizer/humidifier output.

Special Considerations

• Attach heated device to patient only after flow and temperature have stabilized.

TABLE 2-2. HEATERS FOR HUMIDIFIERS AND AEROSOL GENERATORS

TYPE	EXAMPLES	CHARACTERISTICS	ADVANTAGES	DISADVANTAGES
Immersion	Puritan	Rod-shaped electrical heater that extends into the jet nebulizer solution Some models adjustable	Simple to use Relatively inexpensive Solution visible	Hot heater barrel: possible burns Must use separate temperature monitoring and control system Difficult to control temperature Difficult to decontaminate Difficult to service
Wrap-around	Travenol	Wrap-around electric coil that encircles the jet nebulizer, humidifier jar, or stem	Simple to use Relatively inexpensive No need to decontaminate	May become hot to the touch Impossible to see solution in reservoir with wrap-around Cannot control heat Must use separate temperature-monitoring and control system Difficult or impossible to service
Contact pass-over	Ohio Bird Conchatherm	Adjustable heater that attaches to base of jar or allows jet stream to come in contact with heater	Adjustable control No need to decontaminate when element is part of nebulizer or humidifier Solution visible	Expensive Must use separate temperature-monitoring and control system

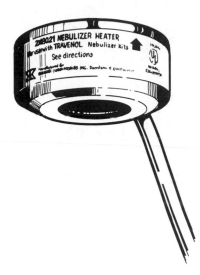

FIG. 2-1. *Nebulizer heater*

- High temperature of solution may result in pulmonary burns.
- Do not use heater with small–bore tubing.
- Always monitor temperature of heated inspired gases.
- Watch tubing for water accumulation.
- Discard water accumulation. (Do not empty back into reservoir.)

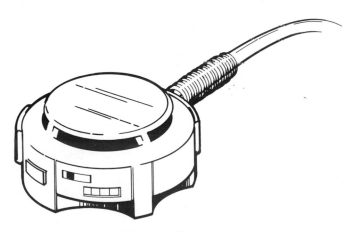

FIG. 2-2. *Base heater*

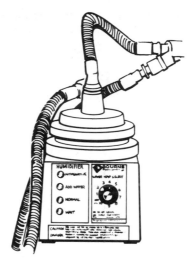

FIG. 2-3. *Humidifier*

- With heaters that are not adjustable, temperature of the inspired gas at the patient outlet may be increased or decreased by varying the tubing length. (Increased tubing length results in decreased temperature; decreased tubing length yields increased temperature.)
- Do not let the reservoir go dry.
- Heated aerosol or humidity may be uncomfortable to the patient who is breathing through his nose or mouth. Adjust temperature for the patient's comfort.
- Heated devices are generally used when the normal humidifying mechanism is bypassed (*i.e.*, when an endotracheal or tracheostomy tube is in place).

Hazards

- Pulmonary burns
- Overmobilization of secretions
- Increased body temperature

Maintenance

- Check electrical plugs for damage.
- Decontaminate immersion heaters following each use.

• Wipe surfaces of all other heaters with a mild cleansing agent followed by a rinse and a decontamination agent, again followed by a rinse.

HEATED VAPORIZER

Description

This large heat-proof reservoir has an immersion-type heater. Water is drawn into a heating column that produces steam (water vapor).

Therapeutic Objective

To decrease a humidity deficit by increasing the relative humidity (water vapor) in a small enclosed area (room).

Criterion for Termination

Relief of humidity deficit

Contraindications

May not provide adequate humidification for most patient needs.

Procedure

1. Fill reservoir with tap water to fill-line.
2. Replace cover.
3. Place vaporizer about four feet from patient. Insert plug into electrical outlet.
4. Steam should be omitted from the vaporizer within 5 to 10 minutes.

Special Considerations

• Place vaporizer in a safe position; the floor is best.
• Do not overfill.
• Use tap water. Mineral content is needed for proper operation.

- If steam is produced too slowly, unplug unit, add 0.25 ml baking soda to water, mix well, and plug unit in again.
- If steam is uneven or produced too rapidly, use half distilled water or clean vaporizer before moving it. Handle with care.

Hazards

- Burns if not handled properly and cautiously
- Steam damage if placed too close to walls
- Shock if cord comes in contact with water

Maintenance

- Clean after each use.
- Rinse unit with bleach and water every five days.
- Remove mineral deposits with distilled white vinegar.

PASS-OVER HUMIDIFIER

Description

This humidifier has a reservoir, a wick, a heater, and housing inlet and outlet ports for tubing connection.

Therapeutic Objective

To humidify inspired gases for either a high- or low-flow oxygen system by passing the gas near a heated wet wick.

Criterion for Termination

Discontinuation of therapeutic gas administration.

Contraindications

None. See Hazards.

Procedure

1. Before assembling the humidifier, insert a wick into the housing.

2. With the wick in place, replace the cap on the bottom of the housing.
3. Attach housing to controller. Replace cap on top of housing.
4. Place humidifier in line with patient.
5. Attach continuous water-feed system; float will maintain constant water level.
6. Make sure humidifier is plugged in.
7. Adjust the heater.
8. Turn on gas flow to warm delivery circuit.
9. Attach set-up to patient.

Special Considerations

• Use continuous feed system.
• System has low gas-flow resistance.
• System has fast warm-up time (less than 5 minutes).
• Monitor inspired gas temperature.
• Built-in high temperature alarm (visual and audible) shuts heater off at 41°C (105°F).
• A remote sensor monitors temperature at proximal airway.
• Provides 100% relative humidity at 37°C.
• Adapts to use with ventilators, oxygen administration systems, tents.
• Used for humidification during neonatal ventilation because of low compliance factor (0.2 ml/cm H_2O).
• No smoking, flames, or ungrounded electrical equipment in area of oxygen use.

Hazards

• Rain-out in tubing occludes the gas flow.
• Malfunction in humidifier controller can cut off heater.
• Minimal potential hazard for transmission of bacteria.

Maintenance

• Keep continuous water-feed system filled and open.
• Monitor temperature at patient wye.

BUBBLE-DIFFUSER HUMIDIFIER (SIMPLE)

Description

This humidifier has a reservoir, a standard connection for a flowmeter, a porous diffuser, and a small-bore outlet connection.

Therapeutic Objective

To humidify inspired gases for low-flow oxygen system by diffusing the gas through water. To prevent loss of water vapor from the respiratory tract.

Criteria for Termination

Discontinuation of therapeutic gas administration. Neutral or positive water balance.

Contraindications

None; however, higher output devices may better meet the patient's needs.

Procedure

1. Fill humidifier reservoir with sterile distilled water.
2. Replace top and attach humidifier to flowmeter.

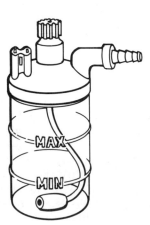

FIG. 2-4. *Bubble humidifier*

3. Turn flow to 3 LPM to check for bubble production. Bubbles should be small and readily apparent.
4. Attach small-bore tubing to humidifier. Connect oxygen-administering device to patient.

Special Considerations

- Pop-off prevents excess pressure build-up when tubing kinks.
- Blockage of small-bore outlet connection cuts off gas flow.
- Small chance of bacteria transfer with this type of unit.
- Provides 20% to 30% relative humidity at 37°C to the patient.
- May be heated to increase relative humidity.
- Can only be used with low-flow devices.
- No smoking, flames, or ungrounded electrical equipment in area of oxygen use.
- Humidifier may be unnecessary with low-flow oxygen (<1.5 LPM).

Hazards

- Inadequate humidity for the patient's needs

Maintenance

- Discard disposable units after use.
- Clean and decontaminate reusable units.
- Keep humidifier filled with sterile distilled water.

BUBBLE-DIFFUSER HUMIDIFIER (CASCADE)

Description

This type of humidifier has a reservoir, a mesh diffuser, large-bore inlet and outlet, and usually an immersion heater.

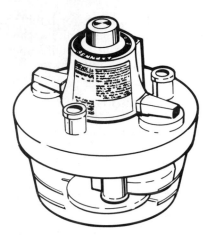

FIG. 2-5. *Cascade humidifier*

Therapeutic Objective

To humidify inspired gases for a high–flow oxygen system by diffusing the gas through heated water. To prevent water loss from respiratory tract.

Criterion for Termination

Discontinuation of therapeutic gas administration.

Contraindications

None. See Hazards.

Procedure

1. Fill humidifier reservoir with sterile distilled water.
2. Replace by screwing jar into cover.
3. Place the cascade in line with patient.
4. Make sure cascade is plugged in, if using heater assembly.

5. Adjust the heater.
6. Allow warm-up time.
7. Turn on gas flow to warm delivery circuit.
8. Attach set-up to patient.

Special Considerations

- Use only sterile water to fill humidifier.
- Temperature of water vapor drops about 2°C per foot of tubing from humidifier.
- Provides 100% relative humidity at 37°C.
- May be Servo-controlled (maintains and sets temperature).
- Warm-up time: 15 to 20 minutes.
- High flow rates/fast ventilator rates = lower temperature.
- Low flow rates/slow ventilator rates = higher temperature.
- Do not permit smoking, flames, or ungrounded electrical equipment in area of oxygen use.

Hazards

- Overheating causes pulmonary burns from dry, hot gas when cascade becomes dry.
- Minimal potential hazard for transmission of bacteria
- Rain-out in tubing may occlude gas flow.
- Inadequate humidification for patient's needs at unheated or low temperatures

Maintenance

- Monitor temperature close to patient wye.
- Do not let fluid level fall below refill-line. Use feed system.
- Check parts for wear (*i.e.*, especially rubber and silicone parts).
- Refill whenever necessary.

TABLE 2-3. HUMIDIFIERS

TYPE	EXAMPLES	HUMIDITY PRODUCED	APPLICATIONS
Heated vaporizer	Hankscraft DeVilbiss	100% RH at 21°C	Increases relative humidity in a small, closed area
Pass-over humidifier	Emerson Ventilator Bird Humidifier	100% RH at 37°C when heated	May be used for large-bore tubing applications or ventilators and high humidity for masks, tents, endotracheal tubes, etc
Bubble diffuser (simple humidifier)	Hudson Travenol American Hospital	40%–50% RH at 21°C (room temperature) 20% RH at 37°C (body temperature)	For use with oxygen-administering devices (e.g., cannula, simple masks). Use where low humidity is adequate for patient's needs. May be unnecessary at very low flow rates
Bubble diffuser (cascade humidifier)	Puritan-Bennett Respiratory Care, Inc.	100% RH at 21°–37°C when heated	Can be used for any large-bore tubing applications or ventilators, CPAP, high humidity with oxygen-enriched systems
Condensing humidifier (heat/moisture exchange)	Siemens Mallinkrodt	70%–90% RH	Filled with hygroscopic medium to collect moisture on exhalation and to warm and humidify on inhalation
Heated wick	Bird Conchapak Fisher and Paykel Travenol	90% RH at 37°C	Gas passed over heated, saturated wick. Adjustable temperature, continuous feed system. Used on ventilator including continuous-flow systems
Vapor phase	Inspiron	90% RH at 37°C when heated	Hydrophobic filter passes water vapor, not liquid. Said to prevent bacteria transmission

ATOMIZER (BULB)

Description

Hand-held aerosol generator uses the squeeze of a bulb to produce a flow of gas. The medication solution is drawn into the flow of gas and a mist is produced (30–100 μ range of particles).

Therapeutic Objectives

To apply a medication locally into the upper airway by generating an aerosol inhaled by the patient.

Criteria for Termination

Relief of bronchospasm, relief of symptoms.

Contraindications

See individual medications (Table 2-4).

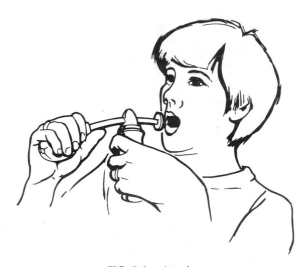

FIG. 2-6. *Atomizer*

TABLE 2-4. AEROSOL MEDICATIONS

MEDICATIONS	EXAMPLE	DOSAGE	INDICATIONS	CONTRA-INDICATIONS	ADVERSE REACTIONS
Bronchodilators					
Albuterol	Ventolin Proventil	1–2 inhalations via metered dose inhaler (MDI) (90 mcg inhalation) q4h Solution: 0.5 ml in 2.5 ml saline 3–4 × day	Relief of bronchospasm Prevention of exercise-induced bronchospasm	Hypersensitivity Do not use other sympathomimetic aerosol bronchodilators at same time	Palpitations, tachycardia, nausea, hypertension, angina, parodoxical bronchoconstriction, vomiting, bad taste
Terbutaline	Brethine	1–2 inhalation MDI (0.20 mg) q4–6h	Relief of bronchospasm	Hypersensitivity	Tachycardia, elevated BP, headache, nausea
Bitolterol Mesylate	Tornalate	2–3 inhalations as treatment (0.37 mg); 2 inhalations q8h as prevention	Relief of bronchospasm Prevention of bronchospasm	Hypersensitivity Do not use other sympathomimetic aerosol or bronchodilators at same time	Tremors, nervousness, headache, palpitations, cough
Isoetharine	Bronkosol	1–2 inhalations MDI (56 mg) Solution: 1% (0.25 ml–1 ml) in saline 3–4 × day	Bronchial dilation Relief of bronchospasm	Hypersensitivity Do not use other sympathomimetic aerosol or bronchodilators at the same time	Tachycardia, nausea, palpitations, restlessness, dry mouth
Isoproterenol	Isuprel	Solution: 1% (0.3 ml) in saline 3–4 × day	Bronchial dilation Relief of bronchospasm		

Drug	Trade name	Dosage	Action	Contraindications/Cautions	Side effects
Metaproterenol	Alupent Metaprel	2–3 inhalations MDI q3–4h (0.65 mg); solution: 0.3 ml in 2.5 ml NaCl 3–4 × day	Bronchodilator	Use in patients with cardiac arrythmias associated with tachycardia	Nervousness, tachycardia, tremor, nausea, hypertension, palpitations, vomiting, bad taste
Epinephrine	Primatene	2 inhalations MDI (0.2 mg) q4h	Temporary relief of acute paroxysms of bronchial asthma	Hypersensitivity Caution with thyroid, high BP, heart disease, diabetes	Bronchial irritation, nervousness, restlessness, sleeplessness
Atropine derivatives		0.1–0.2 ml	Prevents or relieves bronchospasm	Glaucoma Renal failure	Tachycardia, stiffens secretions, dry mouth
Decongestants Phenylephrine	Neo-Synephrine	0.25–1% (0.3–1 ml) in saline 3–4 × day	Reduces edema Vasoconstriction	Hypersensitivity Display of "rebound" effect	Elevated systolic and diastolic blood pressure
Antibiotics Carbenicillin		125–1000 mg in saline 3 × day	Gram-negative bacteria (*Pseudomonas*)	These drugs are of questionable value as an aerosol. Oral routes should be utilized where appropriate.	Bronchospasm Hypersensitivity
Kanamycin		25–300 mg in saline 3 × day	Gram-negative bacteria (*Proteus*)		
Neomycin		25–400 mg in saline 2–4 × day	Gram-negative bacteria (*Staphylococcus/Hemophilus*)		
Polymyxin B		5–50 mg in saline 3–4 × day	Gram-negative bacteria (*Pseudomonas*)		

(Continued)

TABLE 2-4. AEROSOL MEDICATIONS (Continued)

MEDICATIONS	EXAMPLE	DOSAGE	INDICATIONS	CONTRA-INDICATIONS	ADVERSE REACTIONS
Antiasthmatic					
Cromolyn sodium		20 mg × day using a spinhaler or solution for aerosol	Prevents asthma attacks	Hypersensitivity to preparation No role in treatment of acute asthma attack or status asthmaticus	Upper airway irritation, bronchospasm; coughing, nausea, nasal congestion
Mucolytics					
Acetylcysteine	Mucomyst	10% recommended undiluted 20% dilute 1–1 with H_2O or normal saline	Decreases viscosity of mucus	Inhibition of some antibiotics Hypersensitivity to preparation	Bronchospasm, decomposes rubber and metal equipment, expensive
Ethyl alcohol		20%–50%	Pulmonary edema	Alcoholics	Irritation of lung tissue
H_2O			Questionable ability to aid in the liquefaction and mobilization of secretions		Not shown to be therapeutic
$NaHCO_3$		4%–7%	Decreases stickiness of sputum		Breaks down adrenergic bronchodilators
NaCl		0.45%–0.9%–15%	Vehicle for medication delivery	High saline conc. for use in cardiac patients	Sodium retention of fluids

Proteolytics					
Pancreatic dornase		100,000 units in saline 2–3 × day	Purulent secretions	Other mucolytics may be just as effective	Bronchospasm, airway irritation
Steroids					
Beclomethasone	Vanceril	1–2 inhalations MDI (0.042 mg) 3 or 4 × day	Controls asthma attacks Requires chronic treatment with corticosteroids for control of bronchial asthma	Hypersensitivity	Oral infection with *Candida* organism, hoarseness, dry mouth, suppression HPA function
Flunisolide	Aerobid	1–2 inhalation MDI (.25 mg) 2 × day	Requires chronic treatment with corticosteroids for control of bronchial asthma	Hypersensitivity	Vomiting, sore throat
Dexamethasone	Decadron Respihaler	2–3 inhalations (.081 mg) 3–4 × day	Requires chronic treatment with corticosteroids for control of bronchial asthma	Systemic fungal infections Hypersensitivity	*Candida* infections, hoarseness, coughing
Triamcinolone	Azmacort	1–2 inhalations (200 mcg) 3 or 4 × day	Requires chronic treatment with corticosteroids for control of bronchial asthma	In treatment of status asthmaticus and acute episodes of asthma	Hoarseness, dry throat, oral infection with *Candida* organism

Procedure

1. Approach the patient and explain the procedure.
2. Remove the top of the atomizer and place medication solution in the reservoir.
3. Replace top.
4. Have the patient open his mouth and breathe quietly.
5. Instruct the patient to inhale deeply and squeeze the bulb just after the initiation of inspiration.
6. Have the patient hold his breath for 10 to 15 seconds and exhale slowly.
7. Repeat as directed.

Special Considerations

- Used mainly for applying medication to the upper airway.
- Difficult to control dosage.
- Wide range of particle sizes because a baffle is not incorporated.
- Difficult for patient to coordinate breathing cycle and squeezing the bulb.

Hazards

- Local irritation from medication. See specific medication hazards (Table 2-4).

Maintenance

- Clean atomizer following each use.

ATOMIZER (METERED DOSE)

Description

Hand–held aerosol generator that uses a pressurized canister to force the medication through a small jet. Mouthpiece directs medication flow to patient.

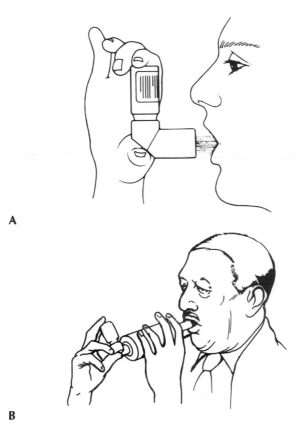

A

B

FIG. 2-7. **A:** *Metered dose inhaler (Bell CW, Blodgett D, Goike CA et al: Home Care and Rehabilitation in Respiratory Medicine, p 219. Philadelphia, JB Lippincott, 1984),* **B:** *Metered dose inhaler with spacer*

Therapeutic Objective

To deliver a metered aerosol dosage of a medication to the patient.

Criteria for Termination

Relief of bronchospasm, relief of symptoms.

Contraindications

Uncoordinated patient. See individual medication.

Procedure

1. Approach the patient and explain the procedure.
2. Attach the mouthpiece to the medication canister. Shake the canister if directed.
3. Direct the patient to place his index finger on top of the canister and his thumb at the bottom of the mouthpiece.
4. Instruct the patient to hold the mouthpiece about 2 inches from his mouth and inhale deeply. Just after the initiation of inspiration, have the patient compress the mouthpiece and canister.
5. Have the patient hold his breath for 10 to 15 seconds and exhale slowly.
6. Repeat as directed.
7. Spacer enhances medication deposition. Attach inhaler to spacer. Shake canister; compress canister and inhale through space.

Special Considerations

• Usually 2 to 3 inhalations 3 to 4 times per day for most bronchodilators. Follow physician's instructions.

Hazards

• Overdosages are possible.
• Specific medication hazards (see Table 2-4).
• Patient coordination of inhaling and squeezing may be inadequate. Use spacer.

Maintenance

• Clean mouthpiece daily to prevent clogging of jet. Clean spacer as necessary.

JET NEBULIZER (LARGE VOLUME)

Description

A jet nebulizer, an atomizer with a baffle, produces an aerosol with a stable particle size (less than 30 μm). A large

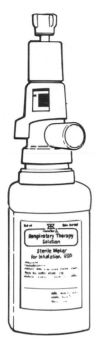

FIG. 2-8. *Nebulizer (large volume)*

jet nebulizer has a reservoir, a gas inlet and outlet, a jet syphon tube, and a system of baffles.

Therapeutic Objective

To provide an output of aerosol (heated or unheated) for intermittent or continuous therapy in order to decrease laryngeal edema, hydrate the respiratory system, and induce a cough to obtain a specimen.

Criteria for Termination

Relief of inspiratory stridor, normal fluid balance.

Contraindication

None. Use caution and monitor patient carefully for hazards.

Procedure

1. Approach the patient and explain the procedure.
2. Fill the nebulizer with sterile distilled water to the fill-line or use prefilled sterile nebulizer.
3. Attach nebulizer to flowmeter.
4. Adjust flow to 12 LPM to check for aerosol production. (FiO_2 depends on source gas and nebulizer entrainment setting.)
5. Attach large-bore tubing to nebulizer.
6. Connect aerosol-administering device to end of large-bore tubing.
7. Set entrainment dial for oxygen concentration.
8. Attach device to patient and adjust flow to keep mist visible.

To vary oxygen concentration:

1. Use blender with 100% source gas.
2. Air gas source with oxygen bled in (low concentration).
3. Oxygen gas source with air bled in (high concentration).

Increased flow is provided by running two nebulizers into wye.

Special Considerations

- Safety relief valve to vent excessive buildup of pressure.
- Dilution control entrains air for desired oxygen concentration.
- May be used heated or unheated.
- Most units should be used with only large-bore tubing. (Puritan All-Purpose can be used on 100% setting with small-bore tubing. Do not use heater with small-bore tubing.)
- Keep jar filled. Do not let unit run dry.
- When water condenses in tubing, drain and discard.
- When using a T-tube, add reservoir tubing to expiration side of T-tube to stabilize oxygen concentration to the patient.
- Monitor FiO_2 when oxygen is used as source gas.
- May be used in line with ventilation devices to provide

heated humidification of inspired gases (Fig. 2-9); however, humidifiers are more appropriate.
- Oxygen concentration can be varied (Fig. 2-10).
- To increase flow, see Figure 2-11.
- May be used on intermittent basis. There are, however, units that produce a better output and range of particle size more appropriate for intermittent use (see Ultrasonic Nebulizer).
- No smoking, flames, or ungrounded electrical equipment in area of oxygen use.

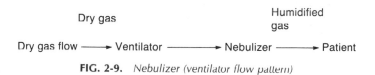

FIG. 2-9. *Nebulizer (ventilator flow pattern)*

Oxygen Concentration can be varied.

    1. Use Blender with 100% Source Gas.
    2. Air Gas source with oxygen bled in (low concentration).
    3. Oxygen Gas source with air bled in (high concentration).

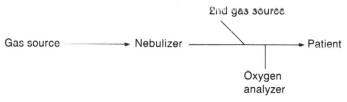

FIG. 2-10. *Nebulizer flow pattern (to vary FIO$_2$)*

Increase Flow can be provided by running two nebulizers into wye.

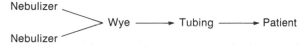

FIG. 2-11. *Nebulizer flow pattern (to increase flow)*

Hazards

- Pulmonary burns with heated unit that overheats or runs dry
- Water accumulation can block gas flow to patient.
- Drying of mucosa when nebulizer runs dry
- Bacterial contamination and transmission. Use humidifiers to humidify inspired gases. Use nebulizers to add liquid volume.

Maintenance

- Replace unit every 24 hours.
- Decontaminate or sterilize after each use.
- Replace worn parts.
- Empty unit before refilling. Rinse and fill with sterile water.

JET NEBULIZER (SMALL VOLUME)

Description

The small-volume jet nebulizer produces an aerosol with a stable range of particle size (less than 30 μm). This device has a small reservoir (less than 20 ml), a gas inlet and outlet, a jet syphon tube, and a baffle system.

Therapeutic Objective

To deposit small amounts of a pharmacologic agent in upper or lower airway.

Criteria for Termination

Relief of bronchospasm, relief of symptoms.

Contraindications

None. See Hazards and specific medications.

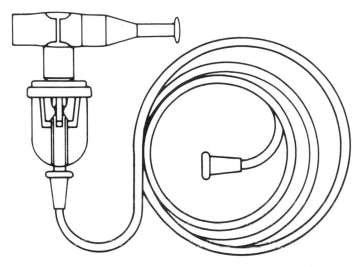

FIG. 2-12. *Nebulizer (small volume) (Bell CW, Blodgett D, Goike CA et al: Home Care and Rehabilitation in Respiratory Medicine, p 217. Philadelphia, JB Lippincott, 1984)*

Procedure

1. Approach the patient and explain the procedure.
2. Attach the nebulizer to the source gas.
3. Fill the nebulizer with the medication prescribed.
4. Turn on the gas flow and adjust nebulizer flow so that a fine mist is visible.
5. Auscultate the chest and monitor vital signs.
6. Instruct the patient to breathe deeply, hold his breath briefly at the end of inspiration, then exhale slowly. Repeat.
7. Instruct the patient to breathe deeply again and cough when necessary to clear the airway.
8. Continue therapy for 10 to 15 minutes or until medication is nebulized. Monitor vital signs and breath sounds.
9. At the completion of the therapy, evaluate the patient for changes in vital signs and breath sounds. Note sputum characteristics.

10. Empty, rinse, and dry nebulizer. Rinse and dry patient appliance.

Special Considerations

- Provide gas in a variety of ways (Fig. 2-13).
- Use only small-bore tubing to power small jet nebulizer.
- Use nebulizer as mainstream or sidestream nebulizer (Fig. 2-14).
- Monitor vital signs, breath sounds, and sputum production before treatment and during and following therapy.
- Nebulizer may be permanent or disposable.
- No smoking, sparks, flames, or ungrounded electrical equipment in area when oxygen is used as source gas.

Hazards

- Bacterial contamination
- Medication side-effects

Maintenance

- Rinse and dry between treatments.
- Exchange nebulizer, tubing, and patient appliance every 24 hours.
- Decontaminate or sterilize after each use. Discard disposables.

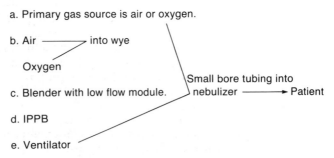

Source gas can be provided in a variety of ways.

a. Primary gas source is air or oxygen.

b. Air ——————→ into wye

Oxygen

c. Blender with low flow module.

Small bore tubing into nebulizer ——————→ Patient

d. IPPB

e. Ventilator

FIG. 2-13. *Nebulizer flow patterns*

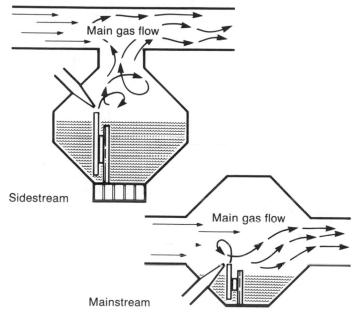

FIG. 2-14. *Nebulizer (sidestream vs. mainstream)*

• Keep the jet clean to maximize output.
• Replace worn parts.

ULTRASONIC NEBULIZER

Description

A solution contained in a chamber vibrates at a high rate, producing a geyser that breaks the solution into very small particles. A flow of gas carries the particles to the patient. This unit has a power source, couplant chamber, nebulizer chamber, and gas-flow inlet and outlet.

Therapeutic Objective

To produce an aerosol with small, stable particles (1–8 μm) to be used intermittently or continuously for aerosol therapy.

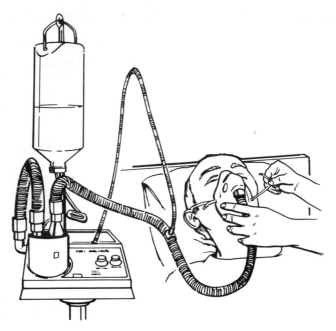

FIG. 2-15. *Ultrasonic nebulizer*

Criteria for Termination

Ability to raise secretions. Clearing of adventitious breath sounds.

Contraindications

Monitor carefully. See Hazards.

Procedure

INTERMITTENT USE

1. Approach the patient and explain the procedure.
2. Place the ultrasonic unit on level surface or use a stand.
3. Plug cord into electrical outlet.
4. Fill couplant chamber with tap water to fill-line.

5. Place nebulizer chamber in couplant chamber and secure.
6. Fill nebulizer chamber to fill-line with sterile solution.
7. Connect nebulizer chamber to gas-flow outlet.
8. Attach large-bore tubing to outlet of nebulizer chamber.
9. Connect other end of large-bore tubing to patient appliance (*i.e.,* aerosol mask, T-tube).
10. Auscultate the chest and monitor vital signs.
11. Place appliance on patient and instruct him to breathe through his mouth.
12. Instruct patient to breathe deeply every few breaths, hold briefly at the end of inspiration, and exhale slowly.
13. Increase output of ultrasonic to level that is easily tolerated by patient.
14. Have the patient breathe deeply and cough.
15. Continue therapy for 10 to 15 minutes. Monitor vital signs and breath sounds throughout treatment session.
16. At the completion of the therapy, evaluate the patient for changes in vital signs and breath sounds. Note sputum production and characteristics.
17. Empty nebulizer chamber; rinse and dry. Rinse and dry patient appliance.

CONTINUOUS USE

1. Approach the patient and explain the procedure.
2. Place the ultrasonic unit on level surface or use a stand.
3. Plug cord into electrical outlet.
4. Fill sterile supply bottle with desired sterile solution (half-normal saline is recommended).
5. Connect feed system to supply bottle.
6. Fill couplant chamber with tap water to fill-line.
7. Place nebulizer chamber in couplant chamber.
8. Attach feed system to nebulizer chamber and allow solution to fill chamber.
9. Attach nebulizer chamber to gas-flow outlet.
10. Attach large-bore tubing to outlet of nebulizer chamber.
11. Connect the large-bore tubing to the patient appliance (face tent, aerosol mask, croupette, mist tent).

12. Turn on generator and adjust to desired level (flush initially for a tent).
13. Position appliance on patient.
14. Evaluate the therapy: Monitor vital signs, breath sounds, and sputum production initially every four hours, and PRN.

Special Considerations

- Monitor FIO_2 when using oxygen.
- Monitor vital signs, breath sounds, and sputum production before treatment and during and after therapy.
- Have suction equipment on hand to clear secretions if necessary.
- For patients who develop bronchospasm, use bronchodilator administration before the therapy when appropriate.
- Daily weights should be obtained on infants and small children receiving continuous ultrasonic therapy.
- Disposable nebulizer chambers are available; some are prefilled.
- Most ultrasonics have an optional drug vial to administer small amounts of medication.
- No smoking, sparks, flames, or ungrounded electrical equipment in area when oxygen is used as source gas.

Use large-bore tubing from nebulizer chamber to patient.

Source gas from:

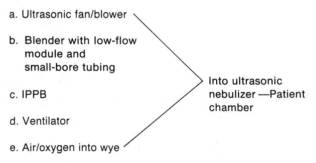

a. Ultrasonic fan/blower

b. Blender with low-flow module and small-bore tubing

c. IPPB

d. Ventilator

e. Air/oxygen into wye

Into ultrasonic nebulizer —Patient chamber

FIG. 2-16. *Ultrasonic flow patterns*

Hazards

- Reflex bronchospasm
- Bacterial contamination
- Fluid overload in infants and small children
- Shocks
- Overmobilization of secretions
- Water accumulation can block gas flow to patient.
- Specific medication hazards (Table 2-4)
- Note: Use continuous ultrasonic therapy with extreme caution.

Maintenance

- Check system frequently to prevent tubing obstruction by water accumulation.
- For continuous use, keep reservoir liquid above fill-line to ensure that nebulizer chamber does not run dry. Use feed system.
- Exchange nebulizer chamber, large-bore tubing, and patient appliance daily and between patients.
- Clean filters between patients and when necessary.

BABBINGTON NEBULIZER

Description

This device uses the hydronamic principle to produce an aerosol with a stable particle size and high output. These units contain a reservoir, aerosol generator, gas inlet and outlet, venturi and filter(s).

Therapeutic Objectives

To humidify inspired gases and to provide a continuous or intermittent output of aerosol.

Criteria for Termination

Ability to raise secretion; decrease in laryngeal edema.

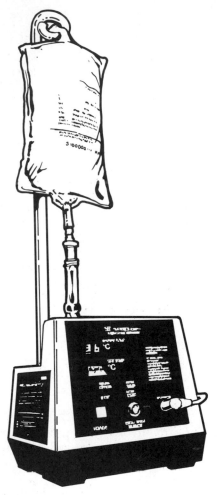

FIG. 2-17. *Servo controlled humidification system*

Contraindications

Use caution; monitor patients for Hazards.

Procedure

See large-volume nebulizer procedure.
See ultrasonic nebulizer procedure.

Special Considerations

- Monitor FiO_2 when oxygen is source gas.
- Output 1 to 7 ml/min 100% relative humidity at BTPS
- Particle size 3–5 μm.
- Monitor vital signs, breath sounds, and sputum production before therapy and during and following therapy.
- No smoking, sparks, flames, or ungrounded electrical equipment when oxygen is used as source gas.

Hazards

- Reflex bronchospasm
- Fluid overload
- Overmobilization of secretions
- Bacterial contamination
- Water accumulation in tubing can block gas flow to patient.

Maintenance

- Check tubing frequently to prevent obstruction in the tubing by water accumulation.
- To ensure that nebulizer chamber does not run dry in continuous use, keep reservoir liquid above fill-line.
- If unit stops misting, lift nebulizer chamber top to eliminate vapor lock. Replace top and unit should start to mist.
- Exchange nebulizer chamber, large-bore tubing, and patient appliance every 24 hours.
- Clean filter daily.

TABLE 2-5. AEROSOL GENERATORS

TYPE	EXAMPLE	AEROSOL/OUTPUT CHARACTERISTICS	APPLICATIONS
Atomizer			
a. Bulb	a. DeVilbiss	a/b. Wide range of particle sizes (30–100 μm), no baffle	Intermittent application of small amounts of medication
b. Metered	b. Ventolin Alupehnt	b. Amount of medication delivered varies depending on manufacturer.	
Centrifugal-spin Disc	DeVilbiss	Wide range of particle sizes and water vapor, 4–8 ml/min output	Room "humidifier"—limited use. Not recommended for hospital use
Jet Nebulizer			
a. Large volume	Puritan All-Purpose Ohio Deluxe Disposable (Travenol)	1–40 range of particle size, 0.5–1 ml/min output, 100% RH at BTPS	Continuous aerosol therapy
b. Small volume	Bird Mironubulizer Puritan Twin Jet	1–40 range of particle size, 0.25–0.5 ml/min output	Intermittent application of small amounts of medication Aerosolization of small amounts of medication
Babbington	Solosphere Maxi-Cool Hydrosphere	3–5 range of particle size for 97% of aerosol produced, 1–7 ml/min output, 100% RH at BTPS	Aerosol therapy (continuous/intermittent)
Ultrasonic	DeVilbiss Mistogen	1–5 range of particle size, 1–6 ml/min output depending on model, 100% RH at BTPS	Aerosol therapy (continuous/intermittent)

84

HEAT AND MOISTURE EXCHANGER

Description

A housing containing hygroscopic material to trap heat and moisture on exhalation. During inhalation, the patient inhales the moisture that was trapped in the exchanger.

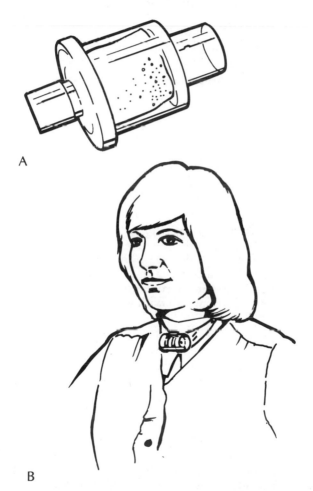

A

B

FIG. 2-18. **A:** *Thermal humidifier;* **B:** *Trach vent*

(70%–90% RH at body temperature under ideal conditions).

Therapeutic Objective

To decrease the humidity deficit.

Criteria for Termination

Discontinuation of inspired dry gases.
Restoration of normal humidification route.

Contraindications

See Hazards

Procedure

1. Follow manufacturer's directions.
2. Insert exchanger between patient and inspired gas generator or attach to artificial airway.

Special Considerations

• Use caution with this device since it may increase airway resistance thereby increasing the work of breathing.
• Check system for mucus contamination.
• Patient may need a system with greater humidity output.

Hazards

• Increased airway resistance
• Blockage
• Inadequate humidity

Maintenance

• Check for blockage.
• Replace disposable inserts as necessary.
• Rinse mucus free with sterile distilled water.

REFERENCES

1. McPherson S: Respiratory Therapy Equipment, p 124. St Louis, CV Mosby, 1985
2. Darin J, Broadwell J, MacDonell R: An evaluation of water-vapor output from four brands of unheated, prefilled bubble humidifiers. Resp Care 27:14–50, 1982
3. Burton GG, Hodgkin JG: Respiratory Care: A Guide to Clinical Practice, 2nd ed. Philadelphia, JB Lippincott, 1984
4. Brain J: Aerosol and humidity therapy. Am Rev Respir Dis 122, No. 5:17–21, 1980

BIBLIOGRAPHY

Ahlgren EW, Chapel JF, Gorgon GI: Pseudomonas aeruginosa infection potential of oxygen humidifier devices. Resp Care 22:383–395, 1977

Brain J: Aerosol and humidity therapy. Am Rev Respir Dis 122, No. 5: 17–21, 1980

Burton GG, Hodgkin JG: Respiratory Care: A Guide to Clinical Practice. Philadelphia, JB Lippincott, 1984

Darin J, Broadwell J, MacDonell R: An evaluation of water-vapor output from four brands of unheated, prefilled bubble humidifiers. Resp Care 27:41–50, 1982

DeKornfeld T: Pharmacology for Respiratory Therapy. Sarasota, Glenn Educational Medical Services, 1976

McFadden ER: Aerosolized bronchodilators and steroids in the treatment of airway obstruction in adults. Am Rev Respir Dis 122, No. 5: 89–96, 1980

McPherson S: Respiratory Therapy Equipment. St Louis, CV Mosby, 1985

Rau J, Rau M: Fundamental Respiratory Therapy Equipment: Principles of Use and Operation. Sarasota, Glenn Educational Medical Services, 1977

Spearman C: Fundamentals of Respiratory Therapy. St Louis, CV Mosby, 1984

Swift D: Aerosols and humidity therapy generation and respiratory deposition of therapeutic aerosols. Am Rev Respir Dis 122, No. 5:71–77, 1980

Wanner A, Rao A: Clinical indications for and effects of bland mucolytic and autimicrobial aerosols. Am Rev Respir Dis 122, No. 5: 79–87, 1980

hyperinflation therapy

Diane Blodgett

Lung expansion for the treatment of atelectasis is one of the respiratory therapist's primary concerns. This chapter examines therapeutic modalities that encourage hyperinflation of the lung, including procedures for rebreathing, incentive spirometry, and intermittent positive pressure breathing (IPPB). Other forms of therapy which may encourage hyperinflation (*e.g.,* breathing exercises, CPAP) are covered in the chapters on chest physiotherapy and assisted ventilation.

In recent years hyperinflation therapy has become a source of controversy in respiratory care. The respiratory care practitioner must at all times evaluate the appropriateness and cost effectiveness of the therapy.

The primary therapeutic objective of hyperinflation therapy is the prevention or treatment of atelectasis in the postoperative or sedentary patient. The development of atelectasis is a risk for patients undergoing thoracic, upper-abdominal, or orthopaedic procedures requiring immobilization. Hyperinflation therapy may benefit them. Also, in some patients, hyperinflation therapy may improve the clearance of secretions from airways. IPPB is not indicated for the delivery of aerosolized medications only since, in this instance, it is no more beneficial than simple aerosol therapy.

The following are general considerations for each generic category of hyperinflation devices.

A. Rebreathing tubes or canisters are employed to increase the patient's deadspace, causing the patient to rebreathe a portion of his exhaled gases. This increases the partial pressure of carbon dioxide contained in the lungs and arterial blood. The response of the body to increased amounts of carbon dioxide in the inspired air varies from individual to individual and even in the same person at different times. Both the central and peripheral chemoreceptors are sensitive to changes in the carbon dioxide tension of the blood. Each set of receptors reacts and triggers an increase in both the depth and rate of ventilation. Because of the varying responses to rebreathing devices, monitor the patient closely. Values as high as 10% to 20% carbon dioxide may be reached with a rebreathing device. Use of this device is contraindicated in patients who are physically unable to increase their tidal and minute ventilation in response to the carbon dioxide. These patients may experience an acute elevation of the arterial carbon dioxide tension and attendant side-effects. Rebreathing devices have limited applications. (See detailed Procedure.)

B. Incentive spirometers, the second major category of hyperinflation devices, encourage the patient to take a maximal sustained inspiration. The process of incentive spirometry, which emphasizes the inspiratory phase of the respiratory cycle, encourages the patient to inhale to maximum capacity. The basic goal of incentive spirometry is the prevention of atelectasis by improving gas distribution. Deep breathing helps to prevent the collapse of alveoli, to reexpand atelectatic areas of the lung, and to stimulate the cough mechanism. Incentive spirometers provide a visual stimulus to encourage the patient as well as a mechanical means of monitoring the patient's progress. Visit the patient often, encourage the patient to perform the maneuvers on his own, and monitor his progress or lack thereof. Minimal hazards exist with this device; however, hyperventilation can occur with an overzealous performer. (See detailed Procedure.) The only real contraindication to the use of the incentive spirometer is the uncooperative patient.

C. Intermittent positive pressure breathing represents the third general category of hyperinflation therapy. IPPB involves administering gas under positive pressure to the airway as a means of increasing the inspired volume. Since the majority of devices used for IPPB are pressure-limited, the volume exhaled should be monitored to assure an increase in tidal volume. Most IPPB machines have a nebulizer which allows the simultaneous administration of

TABLE 3-1. OBJECTIVES AND CRITERIA FOR TERMINATION OF HYPERINFLATION THERAPY

OBJECTIVE	DISEASE AND DISEASE MANIFESTATIONS	TERMINATION
Incentive Spirometry		
1. Treat or prevent atelectasis	Postoperative chest or abdominal case	End of acute postoperative period
2. Assist in deep deposition of aerosol	Asthma	Relief of bronchospasm
		Ability of patient to inhale deeply
		End of acute episode
IPPB		
1. Improve cough	Neuromuscular weakness	Ability to expectorate without assistance
2. Mobilize secretions	Bronchitis	Ability to mobilize and expectorate secretions
3. Treat acute pulmonary edema	Smoke inhalation/cardiac insufficiency	Normal breath sounds
		Return to normal cardiac/respiratory status
4. Improve ventilatory pattern	Postoperative chest or abdominal case	End of acute postoperative period
		Normal breath sounds
5. Decrease work of breathing	Pneumonia	Resolution of pneumonia
		Clear chest x-ray
6. Decrease rising $PaCO_2$	Respiratory insufficiency	Normal ABGs

pharmacologic agents. Supplemental oxygen may also be administered during the IPPB treatment.

IPPB therapy is primarily indicated for patients who are unable to spontaneously increase their tidal volume or are having trouble mobilizing their secretions. In patients with obstructive lung disease, use IPPB with caution in order to prevent an increase in air trapping and possible pneumothorax when the patient coughs. The only absolute contraindication to IPPB is an untreated tension pneumothorax. Associated hazards include hypo- and hyperventilation, decreased cardiac output and pneumothorax, and nosocomial infection. (See detailed Procedure.) Discontinue IPPB when the patient exhibits the ability to (spontaneously) increase his tidal volume and to cough effectively.

Regardless of the hyperinflation therapy employed, quantify the amount of inflation achieved. Assess the overall effectiveness of the therapy by comparing the volume of air exchanged during the therapy to the patient's normal spontaneous ventilation. Unless a significant increase in volume is achieved, the hyperinflation therapy may be of questionable benefit. To assess the need for continued therapy, monitor the patient's total ability in terms of sensorium, muscle strength, caloric intake, etc., as related to his respiratory function. The criterion for termination is the ability of the patient to maintain the integrity of his respiratory function. Evaluate for voluntary lung volumes and flow mechanics, the end of acute post–op period, and clear chest X-rays and auscultatory sounds.

REBREATHING DEVICES

Description

A rebreathing device consists of a cylindrical tube or canister, approximately one liter in volume, with a mouthpiece at one end and an inlet for a supplemental oxygen flow.

Therapeutic Objectives

To increase mechanical deadspace, increase $PaCO_2$, and induce a deep inspiratory maneuver. May be used to treat hysteria and hiccups.

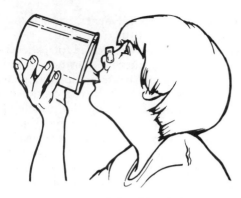

FIG. 3-1. *Rebreathing device*

Criteria for Termination

Calm patient, lack of improvement.

Contraindication

Patients who cannot spontaneously increase their tidal volume or ventilatory rate in response to increased carbon dioxide.

Procedure

1. Approach the patient and explain the procedure.
2. Place patient in semi-Fowler's or sitting position when possible.
3. Place nose clip snugly on patient's nostrils.
4. Have patient breathe normally both into and out through the device. Monitor pulse, blood pressure, and respiration.
5. After five minutes or when the patient's tidal or minute volume has doubled, discontinue the therapy.
6. Monitor patient until rate or volume approach normal resting values.

Special Considerations

- Do not use with patients who, due to weakness or disability, cannot increase their ventilation voluntarily.
- Closely monitor patient's pulse, respirations, and sensorium during therapy.
- Recommended: Monitor the depth and rate of respiration with a spirometer.
- Oxygen or aerosol therapy may be administered during the therapy by entraining aerosol–oxygen mixtures through the device. Oxygen devices that provide a continuous flow through the unit are unacceptable.

Hazards

- Carbon dioxide narcosis (in individuals with chronic respiratory disease), hypercapnia, tachycardia, agitation, cardiac arrhythmia, hypertension, or increased intracranial pressure.

Maintenance

- Exchange the rebreathing device daily to reduce the risk of infection.

□ **INCENTIVE SPIROMETRY**

Description

The incentive spirometer provides visual reinforcement to encourage patients to make a maximal inspiratory effort. The device offers the patient and therapist a means of monitoring progress toward a normal or predetermined goal.

Objective

To encourage patients to take intermittent, spontaneous, maximal inspirations; to prevent or reverse atelectasis, shunting, hypoxia, and hypercarbia; and to aid in deep deposition of aerosol.

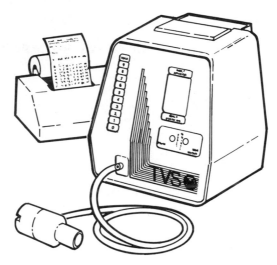

FIG. 3-2. *Incentive spirometer (TVS)*

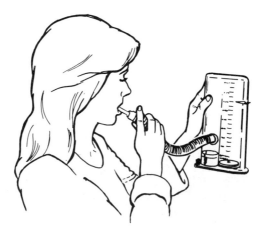

FIG. 3-3. *Incentive spirometer (Voldyne)*

Criteria for Termination

Ability of patient to spontaneously take deep breathes; end of acute post-op period.

Contraindication

Uncooperative patient.

Procedure

1. Approach the patient and explain the procedure.
2. Place the unit in a location convenient for the patient to see and use.
3. Position the patient in an erect, sitting or semi-Fowler's position (whenever possible).
4. Have the patient place the mouthpiece in his mouth and inhale slowly, maintaining a constant flow through the unit. When the patient reaches maximal inspiration he should hold his breath for two to three seconds and then exhale slowly.
5. Following the exhalation, encourage the patient to breathe normally for a short period of time to prevent hyperventilation and exhaustion.
6. Have the patient repeat the maneuver until he reaches the target number of goals.
7. Encourage and coach the patient to cough during the treatment.
8. As patient tolerance improves, increase the volume and number of goals.

Special Considerations

• Aid the patient by splinting incisions.
• Preoperative instruction, including demonstration of diaphragmatic breathing, is desirable for those patients who are likely candidates for postoperative therapy.
• Determination of preoperative capacity aids in determining postoperative goals.
• Locate unit in an area readily accessible to the patient. Encourage use between regular treatment times.

• Patients who are unable to spontaneously initiate a significant inspiratory effort are not good candidates for incentive spirometry.

Hazards

• Hyperventilation and related side-effects.

FLOW-DISPLAYING DEVICES

Description

Lightweight units incorporate an easily visualized indicator inside a flow tube to indicate patient's inspiratory effort.

Considerations for Use

Since the primary goal of incentive spirometry is to have the patient increase his tidal volume (V_T), patients using these devices must suspend the indicator in the flow tube to a determined level for as long as possible. Many of these units provide for the administering of aerosols. The flow from the aerosol generator must be added to the patient's inspired flow in order to estimate true achieved volumes. Maintain the flow-registering tube in an upright position in order to accurately indicate patient effort.

Maintenance

Most units are single-patient devices. Check the unit for free and uniform movement of the flow indicator before use.

VOLUME-DISPLAYING DEVICES

Description

There are two basic categories of volume-displaying units: flow-sensing volume display and volume-displacement devices. The flow-sensing volume display units utilize a flow-registering mouthpiece connected to a volume-display panel. These units require an electrical or battery source and record patient goals as well as volume. The volume-displacement units consist of a piston or bellows contained in a housing. Calibrated indicators display the inspiratory volume achieved by the patient.

Considerations for Use

Do not set patient goals so high that you discourage use. The goals, however, must be high enough to provide a challenge. Carefully select both volume and frequency to encourage the patient to use the device between visits by the therapist. Encourage patients utilizing either type of unit to hold their maximal inspiration for a short period. Not all flow-sensing volume display devices are sensitive enough to indicate small volumes. Readouts may be inaccurate.

Maintenance

Check units regularly for proper function and display. Batteries and light bulbs must be replaced periodically. Monitor current leakage in those units operating on alternating current. Replace mouthpieces daily.

☐ INTERMITTENT POSITIVE PRESSURE BREATHING (IPPB)

Description

IPPB is the short-term (10–20 minutes) delivery of gas with a positive inspiratory pressure, followed by a passive exhalation through the use of a volume-, flow-, or pressure-generating device. Humidity or aerosol therapy can accompany IPPB.

Objectives

To provide a mechanical means of increasing tidal or minute alveolar ventilation, to aid in the prevention and treat-

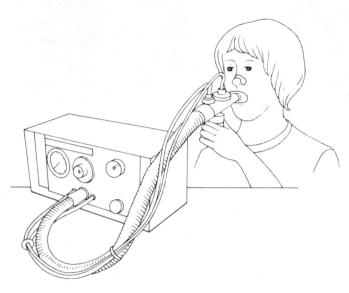

FIG. 3-4. *IPPB AP-5 (Bell CW, Blodgett D, Goike CA et al: Home Care and Rehabilitation in Respiratory Medicine, p 205. Philadelphia, JB Lippincott, 1984)*

ment of atelectasis, hypercapnia and hypoxemia, to reduce temporarily the work of breathing, to mobilize secretions and improve cough, and to treat acute pulmonary edema.

Criteria for Termination

Ability of patient to take spontaneous deep breaths.

Contraindication

Untreated tension pneumothorax.

Procedures

1. Approach patient and explain the procedure.
2. Position the patient in an upright, sitting or semi-Fowler's position if possible.
3. Assemble therapy unit and check for proper function.

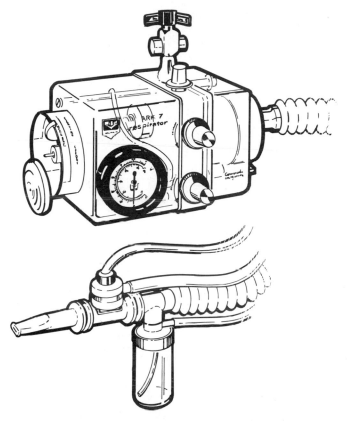

FIG. 3-5. *IPPB Bird*

4. Add medicament to nebulizer, check for proper function. Nebulizer flow should be adequate but not excessive.
5. Determine patient's spontaneous tidal volume or vital capacity as well as pulse, blood pressure, and respiration rate. Auscultate chest.
6. Adjust sensitivity to minimum.
7. If using mouthpiece, place nose clips on patient's nostrils.
8. Initiate treatment using moderate pressures, approximately 15 centimeters of H_2O pressure.

9. Increase pressure and adjust peak-flow controls (if provided) to obtain optimum pressure/flow pattern required to achieve desired tidal volume (10–15 ml/kg).
10. Continue to monitor exhaled tidal volumes during treatment. Reassess the patient throughout the treatment.
11. Continue treatment for specified period of time or until the prescribed medication is delivered.
12. Encourage the patient to cough.
13. Support incisions when required.

Special Considerations

- Maintain an airtight connection between the machine and the patient's airway. Utilize one of a variety of accessories (masks, trach adaptors) available for this purpose.
- Monitor exhaled volumes to assure that the therapeutic goal is achieved.
- Preoperative instruction and demonstration help patients who may require the therapy postoperatively.
- Monitor vital signs throughout therapy.
- Incorporate diaphragmatic and segmental breathing into therapy to achieve optimum expansion of lung segments.

Hazards

- Hazards associated with IPPB include hemoptysis, hypoventilation, hyperventilation, pneumothorax, over-oxygenation, increased intrathoracic pressure with decreased cardiac output, increased intracranial pressure, and gastric insufflation.
- Adverse medication reactions may occur.

Maintenance

- The entire IPPB device should be serviced and calibrated at regular intervals.
- Routine sterilization of the unit may be desirable although not absolutely required with the use of proper bacterial filters.

• Change equipment daily. Rinse and dry nebulizer, mani-
fold, mouthpiece (or mask) following each treatment session.

ELECTRICALLY POWERED AND MANUALLY CYCLED DEVICES

Examples include the Bird Asmastik, Bennett TO and TA
series, Ohio Hand-E-Vent, etc.).

Description

Compact, lightweight units that employ a compressor fitted with a pressure unit (25–30 cm H_2O) and connected to
a nebulizer-exhalation valve-mouthpiece assembly.
Breathing frequency, airway pressure, and tidal volume
are determined by the patient's initiating the closing and
opening of the exhalation valve.

Considerations for Use

These units are specifically designed for home use and do
not offer the flow/pressure capabilities generally required
for intensive therapy. Since the patient controls the inspiratory time and therefore tidal volume, instruct and coach
the patient in the proper technique for increasing tidal volume. Most units employ a venturi to increase the total flow
through the units. As back pressure increases, the flow
from the machine slows. Patients who breathe "against"
the machine and not with it receive smaller tidal volumes
during the same inspiratory time.

ELECTRICALLY POWERED PATIENT-SENSING UNITS

Examples include the Bird Portabird and Bennett AP
series.

Description

Self-contained units consisting of a compressor, an internal pressure regulator, and a patient-sensitive valve for initiating and ending inspiration. These units are fitted with an external patient-supply tube, nebulizer, and exhalation valve.

Considerations for Use

These units combine the portability and ease of operation required for home therapy with the convenience of a patient-assisting or sensing valve. The units may have either a preset or an adjustable limit for pressures achieved, as well as for the effort required to cycle the machine into inspiration. Several also incorporate inspiratory flow-rate controls used to vary the flow of gas to the patient and to regulate the rate of nebulization. In setting the nebulization control, exercise care to prevent diversion of too much of the compressor's output to the nebulizer, thereby decreasing the main flow of gas to the patient.

PNEUMATICALLY POWERED PATIENT-SENSING UNITS

Examples include Bird Mark 7 and 8, Bennett PR, TV, and PV series.

Description

These units, powered by a 50 PSI compressed gas source, may be cycled into inspiration either by patient effort or by a preset timing device. Inspiration generally terminates by achieving a preset pressure, although flow or time may also be a basis for limiting inspiration. Most units provide controls which allow the direct adjustment of inspiratory flow rates. Nebulization is provided through a parallel flow system which, due to the source-gas pressure available, does not effect the mainflow of gas to the patient.

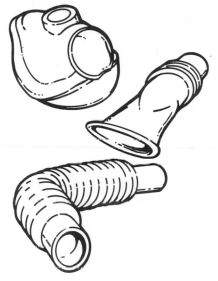

FIG. 3-6. *IPPB accessories*

Considerations for Use

These units are most commonly used in the hospital setting where a standard 50 PSI source of oxygen or air is readily available. When properly applied, the units can increase tidal volumes even in the face of very poor compliance or high resistance. By adjusting the pressure required or the flow rate of the delivered gas, a maximal increase in ventilation with minimal application of positive pressure may be achieved. In order to achieve this goal, carefully titrate pressure and flow rates to each individual patient.

Various accessories (such as masks, trach adaptors) are available to administer therapy.

BIBLIOGRAPHY

Burton GG, Hodgkin JG: Respiratory Care: A Guide to Clinical Practice. Philadelphia, JB Lippincott, 1984
Chase CR et al: Use of a computerized respiratory care record

system to study utilization of IPPB therapy. Resp Care 28, No. 3: 309–314, 1983

Conference on the Scientific Basis of In-Hospital Respiratory Therapy: Mechanical aids to lung expansion. Am Rev Resp Dis 122, No. 5: 23, 105–125, 1980

Demers RR: IPPB treatments: Indications and alternatives. Resp Care 23, No. 1: 758, 1978

Gold M: IPPB therapy, current overview. Resp Care 27, No. 5: 586–587, 1982

Guidelines for the use of intermittent positive pressure breathing (IPPB) prepared by the respiratory care committee of the American Thoracic Society. Resp Care 25, No. 3: 365–370, 1980

Michaeloff M et al: A comparison of intrapulmonary aerosol deposition by IPPB and simple aerosol therapy (abstr). Resp Care 30, No. 10: 882, 1985

Morrison DR, Power WE, Boocks RD: A proposal for the more rational use of IPPB: Volume orientation. Resp Care, 21, No. 3: 318, 1976

O'Donahue W: IPPB past and present. Resp Care 27, No. 5: 588–589, 1982

Shapiro B, Peterson J, Cane R: Complications of mechanical aids to intermittent lung inflation. Resp Care 27, No. 4: 467–470, 1982

Welch MA, Mercurio P, Shapiro B: Letter: The NIH protocol—Is it vulnerable? Resp Care 27: No. 8: 994, 1982

4

chest physiotherapy
Diane Blodgett

This chapter deals with chest physiotherapy procedures, including postural drainage, chest percussion and vibration, rib springing, breathing exercises, and coughing maneuvers. Not all chest physiotherapy procedures are covered here; those that are covered are those generally used in daily respiratory care.

The therapeutic objectives for chest physiotherapy procedures include the removal or prevention of the accumulation of secretions, reexpansion of lung tissue or the prevention of lung tissue collapse, and control of respirations, all of which improve bronchial hygiene and pulmonary function. Physiotherapy procedures may be indicated for both the acute and the chronic respiratory patient. For those patients with retained secretions or collapse of lung tissue, postural drainage or chest percussion and vibration aid in mobilization of secretions and opening of airways. Coughing maneuvers also promote expectoration of sputum and the opening of airways. Breathing exercises benefit patients by decreasing shortness of breath, minimizing oxygen consumption, and decreasing or improving ventilation and muscle utilization.

Contraindications related to postural drainage include active tuberculosis, hemoptysis, untreated pneumothorax, head injury, recent history of cerebral vascular accident, fractured ribs or unstable chest wall, and positional hypotension. Chest percussion, vibration, and rib-springing procedures are contraindicated in patients with empyema, rib fractures, hemoptysis, lung tumors, pain, and fragile bony structures. There are no apparent contraindications to breathing exercises and there are really only precautions for coughing maneuvers. With the patient who has an incision, for example, care must be taken to guard against pain and stress on the incision site when coughing.

The criteria for termination of chest physiotherapy are a clear chest x-ray, normal ausculatory sounds, the ability to mobilize secretions, and/or the ability to normalize and control the breathing pattern.

POSTURAL DRAINAGE

Description

Postural drainage is the positioning of the patient to drain various lung segments.

Therapeutic Objective

To facilitate drainage and removal of secretions from the lung by taking advantage of gravitational forces.

Criteria for Termination

Normal ausculatory sounds, clear chest x-ray, normal ability to clear secretions.

Contraindications

Active tuberculosis, hemoptysis, untreated pneumothorax, head injury, recent CVA, positional hypotension, fractured ribs, unstable chest wall.

Procedure

1. Approach the patient and explain the procedure.
2. Place the patient in proper position for drainage of specific lobe or segment.
3. Leave the patient in this position for at least 15 to 20 minutes.
4. During this time period have the patient breathe deeply and cough.

5. Return the patient to the sitting position and ask him to breathe deeply and cough.

Special Considerations

- Monitor vital signs (HR, RR, BP).
- Make sure the patient is comfortable
- Support the patient's position with the use of pillows and bed rolls.
- Provide the patient with tissues and sputum cup for expectorated secretions.
- Have suction equipment available to remove secretions that may accumulate in the airway.
- Reduce the time of drainage when percussion is used in conjunction with postural drainage.
- Do not attempt drainage immediately following a meal.
- Monitor vital signs carefully, especially in the head-down position.
- Use breathing exercises and coughing maneuvers to facilitate loosening of secretions.
- Give any adjunct therapy, such as aerosol, IPPB, or ultrasonic therapy (USN) before chest physiotherapy.
- For patients who have generalized disease, start with the lower lobes, then clear the middle lobes, and finally the upper lobes. For small children, start with the upper lobes, then the middle lobes, and finally the lower lobes. For patients with localized disease, start with the involved segment, and then the segments that are disease-free.

Hazards

- Positional hypotension
- Increasing dyspnea
- Overmobilization of secretions
- Tipping may lead to further collapse in untreated pneumothorax.
- Increased intracranial pressure
- Hypoxemia

Maintenance

- Keep the patient comfortable during procedure.

CHEST PERCUSSION (CLAPPING, CUPPING, TAPPING)

Description

Chest percussion uses the hands in the cupping, clapping, or tapping position to set up vibrations over various segments of the chest wall.

Therapeutic Objective

To loosen and aid in the removal of lung secretions to promote reexpansion of lung tissue and augment postural drainage.

Criteria for Termination

Clear chest x-ray film, normal breath sounds, ability of patient to mobilize his secretions.

Contraindications

Untreated pneumothorax, active pulmonary hemorrhage, large lung abscess or effusion, status asthmaticus, acute postoperative neurosurgery.

Procedure

1. Approach the patient and explain the procedure.
2. Since this procedure is almost always used in conjunction with postural drainage, place the patient in the proper position for drainage of a specific lobe or segment (see Tables 4-1, 4-2).
3. Position hands for cupping, clapping, or tapping over indicated area for each segment to be drained and percuss for 3 to 5 minutes.
4. After each position, have the patient breathe deeply and cough.
5. Return the patient to the sitting position and again ask him to cough.

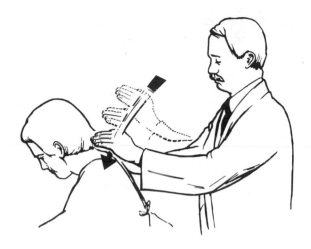

A

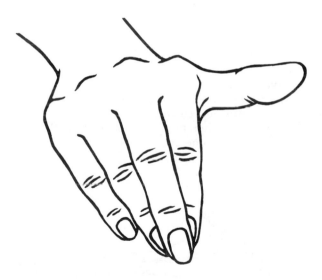

B

FIG. 4-1A: *Chest percussion: Clapping (cupping);* **B:** *Chest percussion: Hand position (Blodgett D: Manual of Pediatric Respiratory Care Procedures, p 65. Philadelphia, JB Lippincott, 1982)*

TABLE 4-1. GENERAL POSITIONS AND INSTRUCTIONS FOR CHEST PHYSICAL THERAPY

UPPER LOBES APICAL (FIG. 4-2)	Percuss and vibrate over uppermost portion of both sides of the chest to the nipple.
UPPER LOBES POSTERIOR (FIG. 4-3)	Percuss and vibrate over posterior scapular area on both sides
LEFT LOWER LOBE AND LINGULA (FIG. 4-4)	Percuss and vibrate left side and back from axilla to bottom of ribs.
RIGHT MIDDLE & LOWER LOBE (FIG. 4-5)	Percuss and vibrate right side and back from axilla to bottom of ribs.
LOWER LOBES (FIG. 4-6)	Percuss and vibrate either side of vertebra from scapula to bottom of ribs.

Special Considerations

- Monitor vital signs (HR, RR, BP).
- Make sure the patient is comfortable.
- Use rhythmic percussion.
- Adjust amount of force to the individual patient but do not use forceful movements.
- Give any adjunct therapy, such as aerosol, IPPB, or USN before chest physiotherapy.

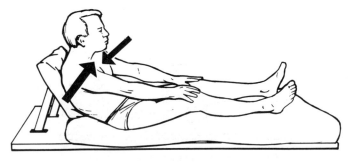

FIG. 4-2. *Upper lobes (apical). Patient sitting in upright position. Percuss and vibrate over uppermost portion of both sides of the chest to the nipple.*

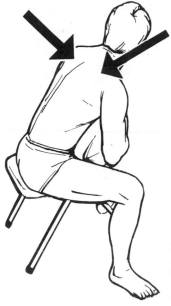

FIG. 4-3. *Upper lobes (posterior). Patient sitting and leaning forward with pillow in abdominal area. Percuss and vibrate over posterior scapular area on both sides.*

- Do not percuss on bare skin.
- Do not percuss over kidneys, spine, or female breasts.
- Give any ordered pain medication before chest physiotherapy to lessen discomfort.
- Do not percuss over area of tuberculosis, empyema, or cancerous tumors.

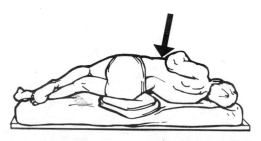

FIG. 4-4. *Left lower lobe and lingula. Patient lying on right side with head down or pillow under hips. Percuss and vibrate left side and back from axilla to bottom of ribs.*

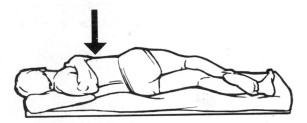

FIG. 4-5. *Right middle and lower lobe. Patient lying on left side with head down or pillow under hips. Percuss and vibrate right side and back from axilla to bottom of ribs.*

- Observe the same special considerations as for postural drainage.
- Do not percuss over drainage tubes.

Hazards

- Increased bronchospasm in asthmatics
- Fractured ribs
- May spread infection or tumor
- May increase pulmonic bleeding or cause overmobilization of secretions
- Note other hazards under Postural Drainage.

Maintenance

- Keep the patient comfortable during the procedure.

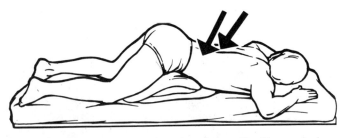

FIG. 4-6. *Lower lobes. Patient lying face down with pillow under lower chest and abdominal area. Percuss and vibrate either side of vertebra from scapula to bottom of ribs.*

TABLE 4-2. POSITIONS AND INSTRUCTIONS FOR DRAINAGE OF SPECIFIC LUNG SEGMENTS

RUL APICAL (FIG. 4-7)	Percuss and vibrate over uppermost portion of right back area.
RUL ANTERIOR (FIG. 4-8)	Percuss and vibrate over upper third of right side of chest.
RUL POSTERIOR (FIG. 4-9)	Percuss and vibrate over upper third of ribs on right side of back.
RML LATERAL MEDIAL (FIG. 4-10)	Percuss and vibrate over right nipple area.
RLL SUPERIOR (FIG. 4-11)	Percuss and vibrate over middle third of ribs on right back.
RLL MEDIAL BASAL (FIG. 4-12)	Difficult to percuss over appropriate area.
RLL ANTERIOR BASAL (FIG. 4-13)	Percuss and vibrate over lower third of ribs on right side below the axilla.
RLL LATERAL BASAL (FIG. 4-14)	Percuss and vibrate over middle third of ribs on right side.
RLL POSTERIOR BASAL (FIG. 4-15)	Percuss and vibrate over lower third of ribs on right back.
LUL APICAL POSTERIOR (FIG. 4-16)	Percuss and vibrate over uppermost portion of left back.
LUL ANTERIOR (FIG. 4-17)	Percuss and vibrate over upper third of left side of chest.
LUL LINGULA INFERIOR-SUPERIOR (FIG. 4-18)	Percuss and vibrate over middle third of ribs on left back.
LLL SUPERIOR (FIG. 4-19)	Percuss and vibrate over middle third of ribs on left back.
LLL ANTERIOR BASAL (FIG. 4-20)	Percuss and vibrate over lower third of ribs on left side below the axilla.
LLL LATERAL BASAL (FIG. 4-21)	Percuss and vibrate over middle third of ribs on left side.
LLL POSTERIOR BASAL (FIG. 4-22)	Percuss and vibrate over lower third of ribs on left side.

Figures 4-7 through 4-22 are from Blodgett D: Manual of Pediatric Respiratory Care Procedures, pp 56–60. Philadelphia, JB Lippincott, 1982

(*Text continues on p. 122.*)

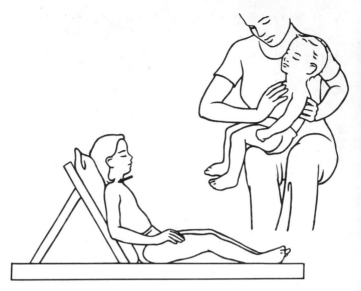

FIG. 4-7. *Right upper lobe (apical). Patient lying on back. Head raised to 30° angle. Percuss and vibrate over uppermost portion of right back area.*

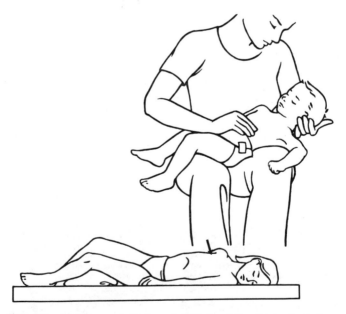

FIG. 4-8. *Right upper lobe (anterior). Patient lying flat on back, knees supported. Percuss and vibrate over upper third of right side of chest.*

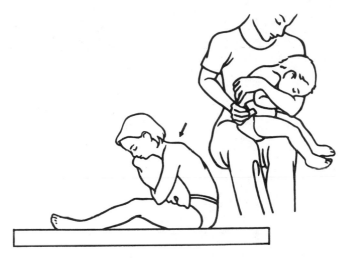

FIG. 4-9. *Right upper lobe (posterior). Patient sitting and leaning forward with pillow in abdominal area. Percuss and vibrate over upper third of ribs on right side of back.*

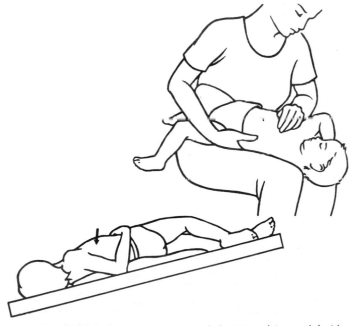

FIG. 4-10. *Right middle lobe (lateral medial). Patient lying on left side with head down, right side back ¼ turn, knees flexed. Percuss and vibrate over right nipple area.*

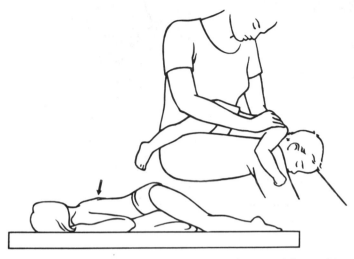

FIG. 4-11. *Right lower lobe (superior). Patient lying on abdomen, hips supported. Percuss and vibrate over middle third of ribs on right back.*

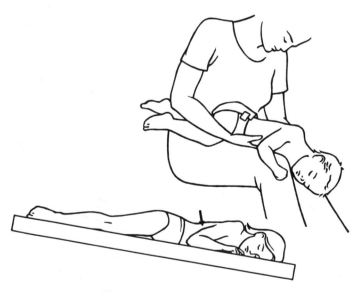

FIG. 4-12. *Right lower lobe (medial basal). Patient lying on abdomen with head down, hips supported, left side turned up slightly. Difficult to percuss over appropriate area.*

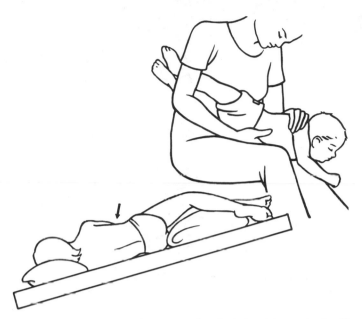

FIG. 4-13. *Right lower lobe (anterior basal). Patient lying on back with head down, knees supported. Percuss and vibrate over lower third of ribs on right side below the axilla.*

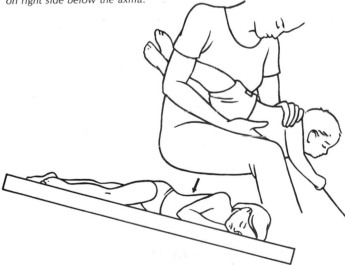

FIG. 4-14. *Right lower lobe (lateral basal). Patient lying on abdomen with head down, right side turned up slightly, hips supported. Percuss and vibrate over middle third of ribs on right side.*

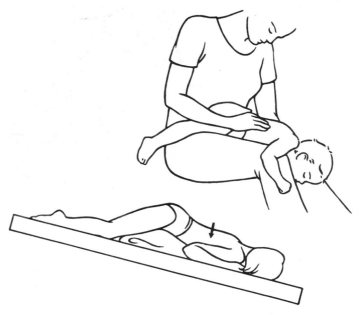

FIG. 4-15. *Right lower lobe (posterior basal). Patient lying on abdomen in head-down position, hips supported. Percuss and vibrate over lower third of ribs on right back.*

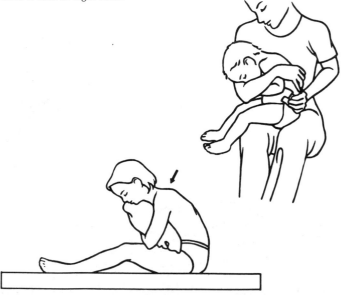

FIG. 4-16. *Left upper lobe (apical posterior). Patient lying on back, head raised to 30°. Percuss and vibrate over uppermost portion of left back.*

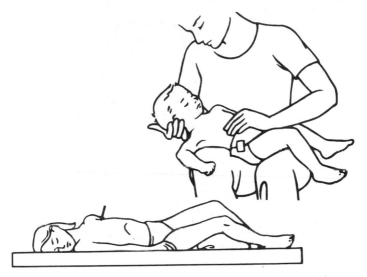

FIG. 4-17. *Left upper lobe (anterior). Patient lying flat on back, knees supported. Percuss and vibrate over upper third of left side of chest.*

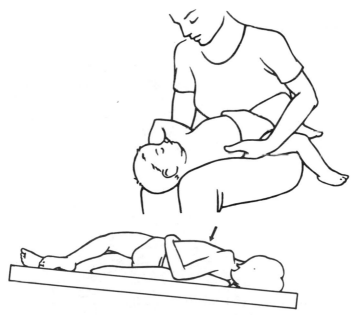

FIG. 4-18. *Left upper lobe (lingula inferior–superior). Patient lying on right side with head down, left side back ¼ turn, knees flexed. Percuss and vibrate over middle third of ribs on left back.*

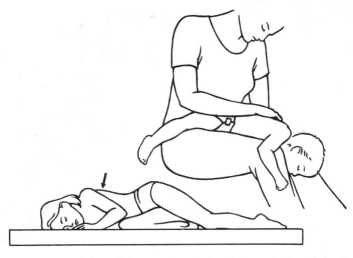

FIG. 4-19. *Left lower lobe (superior). Patient lying on back with head down, knees supported. Percuss and vibrate over lower third of ribs on left side below the axilla.*

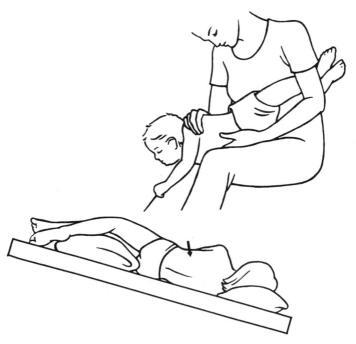

FIG. 4-20. *Left lower lobe (anterior basal). Patient lying on abdomen with left side turned up slightly, hips supported. Percuss and vibrate over middle third of ribs on left side.*

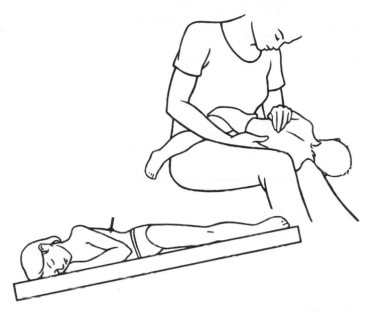

FIG. 4-21. *Left lower lobe (lateral basal). Patient lying on abdomen in head-down position, hips supported. Percuss and vibrate over lower third of ribs on left side.*

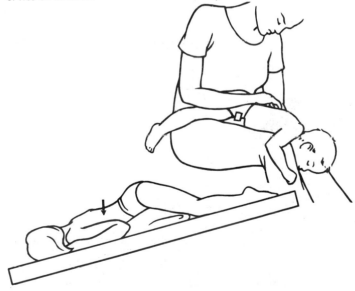

FIG. 4-22. *Left lower lobe (posterior basal). Patient lying prone over pillow, hips supported. Percuss and vibrate over middle third of ribs on left back.*

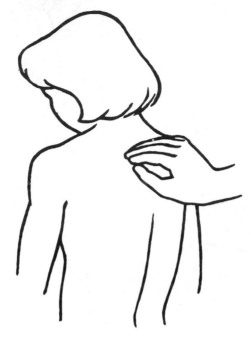

FIG. 4-23. *Chest percussion: Tapping (Blodgett D: Manual of Pediatric Respiratory Care Procedures, p 64. Philadelphia, JB Lippincott, 1982)*

CHEST VIBRATION

Description

Chest vibration is the placing of flat hands over area to be drained and vibrating the hands quickly during the expiratory phase of the respiratory cycle.

Therapeutic Objective

Aids in the loosening of secretions and the mobilization of secretions toward the trachea.

Criteria for Termination

Clear chest x-ray film, normal ausculatory sounds, ability of patient to mobilize his secretions.

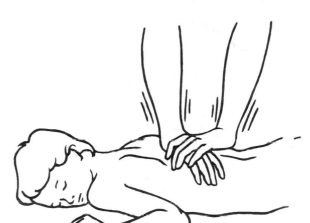

FIG. 4-24. *Chest percussion; Vibration (Blodgett D: Manual of Pediatric Respiratory Care Procedures, p 66. Philadelphia, JB Lippincott, 1982)*

Contraindications

Hemoptysis, displaced rib fractures.

Procedure

1. Approach the patient and explain the procedure.
2. Since this procedure is almost always used in conjunction with postural drainage, place the patient in the proper position for drainage of a specific lobe or segment (see Tables 4-1, 4-2).
3. Place the flat of the hands over the area to be vibrated.
4. As the patient exhales, press firmly against the chest wall area; the contractions of the arm and shoulder muscle create vibrations in the hands.
5. Vibrate for 3 to 5 minutes over each segment as indicated.
6. After each position, have the patient breathe deeply and cough.
7. Return patient to sitting position and again ask him to breathe deeply and cough.

Special Considerations

- Monitor vital signs (HR, RR, BP).
- Do vibration only during expiration.
- Vibrate from the top of inspiration to end of expiration.
- Give any adjunct therapy, such as aerosol, IPPB, or USN before chest therapy.
- Do not vibrate over area of tuberculosis, empyema, or cancerous tumor.
- Give pain medication before chest therapy to lessen discomfort.
- Do not vibrate on bare skin.
- Observe special considerations for postural drainage.

Hazards

- Increased bronchospasm in asthmatics
- May spread infection or tumor
- Note other hazards under Postural Drainage.

Maintenance

- Keep the patient comfortable during the procedure.

RIB SPRINGING

Description

Rib springing is a maneuver that puts intermittent pressure on the chest wall during the expiratory phase.

Therapeutic Objective

Aids in loosening and transporting secretions in the direction of the trachea.

Criteria for Termination

Clear chest x-ray film, normal breath sounds, ability of patient to mobilize his secretions.

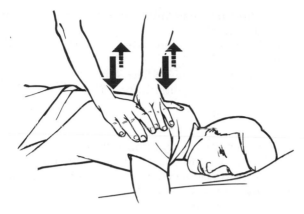

FIG. 4-25. *Chest percussion rib springing*

Contraindications

Fractured ribs, untreated pneumothorax, active pulmonary hemorrhage, large lung abscess or effusion, status asthmaticus.

Procedure

1. Approach the patient and explain the procedure.
2. Since the procedure is almost always used in conjunction with postural drainage, place the patient in the proper position for drainage of a specific lobe or segment.
3. Place the flat of the hands over the area to be drained.
4. As the patient exhales, exert pressure and relax pressure 3 to 4 times with a springlike action.
5. Repeat every other breath for one minute.
6. After each position, have the patient breathe deeply and cough.
7. Return patient to sitting position and again ask him to cough.

Special Considerations

- Monitor vital signs (HR, RR, BP).
- Give any adjunct therapy such as aerosol, IPPB, or USN before chest therapy.

- Do not use pressure over area of tuberculosis, empyema, or cancerous tumor.
- Give pain medication before chest therapy to lessen discomfort.
- Do not use rib springing on bare skin.
- Observe special considerations for postural drainage.

Hazards

- Increased bronchospasm in asthmatics
- Do not use on patients with immobile chest wall (*i.e.,* patient with emphysema or increased A–P diameter).
- May increase pain in post-op thoracic patient
- Note other hazards under Postural Drainage.

Maintenance

- Keep the patient comfortable during the procedure.

BREATHING EXERCISES

Description

Breathing exercises incorporate techniques to help the patient control the volume and flow of air into and out of the lungs.

Therapeutic Objectives

To normalize the pattern of breathing, improve ventilation, foster relaxation, decrease oxygen consumption, decrease work of breathing, and encourage relaxation.

Criteria for Termination

Normal breathing pattern, ability of patient to control breathing pattern.

Contraindications

Severe pain, uncooperative patient.

Procedure

DIAPHRAGMATIC BREATHING

1. Approach the patient and explain the procedure.
2. Position the patient in the supine position with the knees bent and feet flat. Have the patient place one of his hands on his chest and one on his abdomen.
3. Instruct the patient to push his abdomen out against his hand as he inhales. Demonstrate procedure.
4. Direct the patient to pull his abdomen in as he exhales.
5. Have him repeat this at a slightly slower-than-normal breathing rate. Repeat 10 times.
6. When the patient has mastered the exercise in the supine position, instruct him to follow the same procedure in the sitting and standing positions.

Special Considerations
- Monitor vital signs.
- Weights may be placed on the diaphragm to increase muscle strength.
- Use this procedure in combination with pursed-lip breathing.

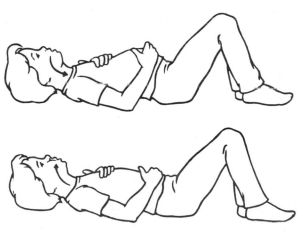

FIG. 4-26. *Diaphragmatic breathing (supine) (Blodgett D: Manual of Pediatric Respiratory Care Procedures, p 71. Philadelphia, JB Lippincott, 1982)*

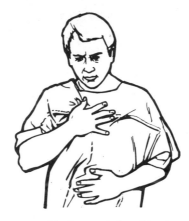

FIG. 4-27. *Diaphragmatic breathing (standing)*

• Belt may be used instead of hand pressure. Loose ends of belt are pulled tight during expiration.

PURSED-LIP BREATHING

1. Approach the patient and explain the procedure.
2. Demonstrate the technique.
3. Place the patient in a relaxed sitting or supine position.
4. Guide the patient through the breathing cycle.
5. Instruct the patient to take a normal inspiration through his nose.
6. Direct the patient to purse his lips and exhale.
7. Have the patient slow his exhalation, but do not allow him to prolong the expiratory phase extensively.
8. Repeat.

Special Considerations

• Monitor vital signs.
• Have the patient exhale against resistance by placing three fingers lightly over his mouth.
• Use this procedure in combination with diaphragmatic breathing.
• Have patient try to blow out candle while using pursed lip breathing.

SEGMENTAL (COSTAL) BREATHING

1. Approach the patient and explain the procedure.
2. Demonstrate the procedure.

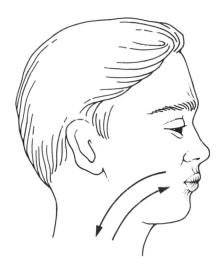

FIG. 4-28. *Pursed-lip breathing (Bell CW, Blodgett D, Goike CA et al: Home Care and Rehabilitation in Respiratory Medicine, p 159. Philadelphia, JB Lippincott, 1984)*

3. Place your hand over the affected area of the lung.
4. Instruct the patient to inhale slowly while pushing out against his hands.
5. Exert pressure on the affected area as the patient exhales.
6. Repeat.
7. Have the patient place his hand over the area and follow this procedure.
8. Repeat 10 times.

Special Considerations
- Monitor vital signs.
- This technique is quite difficult for some patients to do.
- As the patient inhales, keep hand lightly on affected area.
- Patient must be cooperative and understand the instructions.

General Considerations
- All exercises should be taught in a quiet, calm atmosphere.
- Make sure the patient is comfortable.
- Use many positions (sitting, standing, reclining, walking) to teach the exercises.

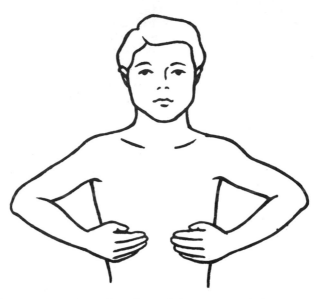

FIG. 4-29. *Lateral costal breathing (Blodgett D: Manual of Pediatric Respiratory Care Procedures, p 72. Philadelphia, JB Lippincott, 1982)*

- Discourage patient from using accessory muscles.
- Use breathing exercises in conjunction with other types of respiratory care when indicated.
- Have patient keep correct posture during exercise to facilitate full lung expansion.
- Give encouragement and reinforcement to all patients while they are learning these techniques.

Hazards

- Overexertion and fatigue when the patient forces the exercises
- Increasing shortness of breath when patient attempts to do exercises rapidly
- Hyperventilation

Maintenance

- Coach the patient many times to ensure that the exercises are being done correctly.

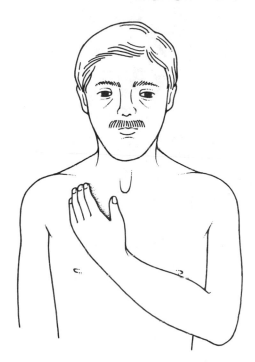

FIG. 4-30. *Segmental breathing (Bell CW, Blodgett D, Goike CA et al: Home Care and Rehabilitation in Respiratory Medicine, p 161. Philadelphia, JB Lippincott, 1984)*

COUGHING MANEUVERS

Description

Coughing consists of a deep inhalation, closure of the glottis, contraction of respiratory muscles, the opening of the glottis, and rapid expulsion of air.

Therapeutic Objective

Promotes expansion of lung tissue and mobilizes and clears the airway of secretions.

Criteria for Termination

None.

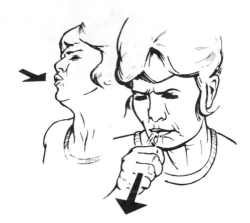

FIG. 4-31. *Coughing*

Contraindications

There is no real contraindication to coughing, only to explosive, forceful coughing.

Procedure

1. Approach the patient and explain the procedure.
2. Position the patient for maximum effectiveness of maneuver; for most patients sitting is best, while for patients with respiratory muscle impairment the head-down position is better.
3. Instruct the patient to take in a slow, deep breath and hold it.
4. Instruct the patient to contract the abdominal muscle and exhale rapidly while contracting his throat muscles.
5. Have the patient follow this pattern:
   Inhale—Hold—Contract muscles
   Exhale (small amount)—Cough—Exhale (small amount)
6. Repeat

Special Considerations

- Splint patients with incision or pain.
- Give pain medication before respiratory therapy to decrease discomfort.

- For those patients who cannot take a deep breath, the therapist should augment the attempt with assisted ventilation (IPPB, manual resuscitator).
- For those patients who cannot exhale forcibly, the therapist should place hands on the diaphragm and push during exhalation.
- Have the patient say "K, K, K" during contraction of the throat muscles to assist the coughing effort.

Hazards

- Do not make the patient cough too long or hard.
- Venous return may be impaired.
- Precautions should be taken with those patients who have vascular abnormalities (CVA, aneurysms, etc.).
- Asthmatics may increase bronchospasm in hyperactive airways.
- Uncontrollable coughing spasms may aggravate symptoms.

CONDITIONING EXERCISES

Description

Exercise promotes the physical and mental well-being of the patient. Specific exercises address such problems as chest immobility and postural defects.

Therapeutic Objective

Improve posture, increase upper chest mobility.

Criteria for Termination

Improvement in posture and chest mobility.

Contraindications

Uncooperative patients, patients with generalized weakness.

Procedure

POSTURE: PATIENT INSTRUCTIONS

1. Stand against wall with feet about 4 inches from support.
2. Bend down while exhaling using your abdominal muscles.
3. Raise yourself as you push your spine progressively against the wall. Start inhaling during this maneuver.
4. Press your lower back against wall and relax. Continue to inhale slowly.
5. Complete inspiration using your diaphragm.

MOBILITY: PATIENT INSTRUCTIONS

(A) 1. Stand up using good posture.
    2. Allow your arms to swing loosely while turning at the waist from side to side.

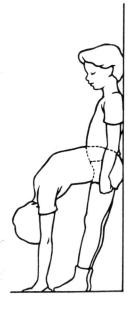

FIG. 4-32. *Posture (Blodgett D: Manual of Pediatric Respiratory Care Procedures, p 77. Philadelphia, JB Lippincott, 1982)*

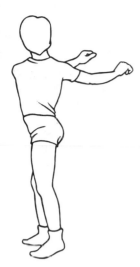

FIG. 4-33. *Mobility (Blodgett D: Manual of Pediatric Respiratory Care Procedures, p 78. Philadelphia, JB Lippincott, 1982)*

(B) 1. Stand using good posture.
2. Alternately swing arms in a circle like a windmill.
(C) 1. Stand using good posture.
2. Extend your arms straight out in front of you.
3. Take a deep breath and exhale.
4. Return arms to your side.
5. Extend your arms straight out to the side.
6. Take a deep breath and exhale.
7. Return arms to your sides.
8. Put arms behind your back. Stretch.
9. Breathe deeply, relax, exhale.

Hazards

Falls with unstable patients

Special Considerations

- Have patient repeat exercises 2 to 3 times a day in 15-minute sessions.
- Do not fatigue the patient. Weaker patients may require shorter sessions.

RELAXATION TECHNIQUES

Description

Relaxation techniques promote relaxation of the chest wall, neck, and abdominal muscles, and help to decrease anxiety.

Therapeutic Objective

To slow respiratory rate, decrease work of breathing, decrease oxygen consumption, improve gas exchange.

Criterion for Termination

Decrease in stress factors.

Contraindications

None.

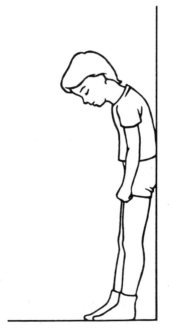

FIG. 4-34. *Relaxation (standing position) (Blodgett D: Manual of Pediatric Respiratory Care Procedures, p 80. Philadelphia, JB Lippincott, 1982)*

Procedure

RELAXATION POSITIONS: PATIENT INSTRUCTIONS

(A) 1. Standing: Place your feet about 6 to 8 inches from the wall.
    2. Lean back against the wall. Let your arms hang loosely at your side.
(B) 1. Sitting: Place your feet flat on floor. Sit with your elbows on your thighs.
    2. Relax the muscles of the shoulders and neck. Breathe slowly; do not force respirations.

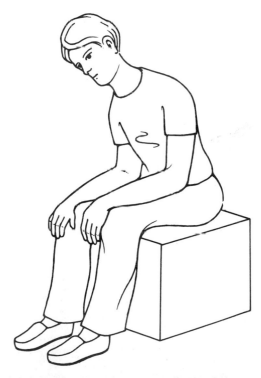

FIG. 4-35. *Relaxation (sitting position) (Bell CW, Blodgett D, Goike CA et al: Home Care and Rehabilitation in Respiratory Medicine, p 171. Philadelphia, JB Lippincott, 1984)*

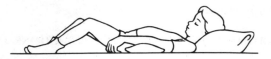

FIG. 4-36. *Relaxation (supine) (Blodgett D: Manual of Pediatric Respiratory Care Procedures, p 81. Philadelphia, JB Lippincott, 1982)*

(C) 1. Supine: Lay on the bed with your head supported with a pillow.
   2. Place pillow under each arm for support. Flex the knees slightly and breathe slowly.

RELAXATION TECHNIQUES: PATIENT INSTRUCTIONS

(A) 1. Place yourself in a relaxed position either sitting or lying.
   2. Close your eyes.
   3. Concentrate on slow, controlled breathing.
   4. Tense the muscle groups in your face (nose, eyes). Hold for 2 seconds and release.
   5. Tense your neck and shoulder muscles. Hold and release.

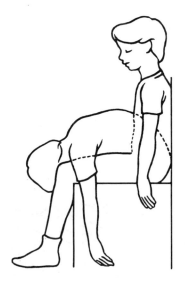

FIG. 4-37. *Relaxation techniques (Blodgett D: Manual of Pediatric Respiratory Care Procedures, p 81. Philadelphia, JB Lippincott, 1982)*

6. Tense your hand and arm muscles. Hold and release.
7. Tense your chest and abdominal muscles. Hold and release.
8. Tense your feet and leg muscles. Hold and release.
9. Relax. Concentrate on how your muscles feel now that the muscles are relaxed.

(B) 1. Place yourself in a sitting position, arms hanging at your side.
2. Breathe out slowly while dropping your head.
3. Bend forward until your head is between your legs.
4. Tighten your abdominal muscles.
5. Breathe in slowly while returning to the sitting position.
6. Move hips, the back, shoulders, and finally neck to sitting position.

Special Considerations

- Provide patient encouragement throughout the initial learning session.
- Teach techniques in a quiet, calm atmosphere. Room should have subdued lighting and the instructor should have a calm, reassuring voice.
- Have patient practice techniques at least once a day. Best time is at bedtime.
- Have patient perform techniques and use positions whenever dyspnea or tenseness appears or when the patient wishes to relax.
- Encourage patient to remain calm during stressful situations, especially during periods of dyspnea.

RESPIRATORY MUSCLE TRAINING

Description

Respiratory muscle training uses either inspiratory resistive breathing or isocapnic hyperpnea to exercise the ventilatory musculature.

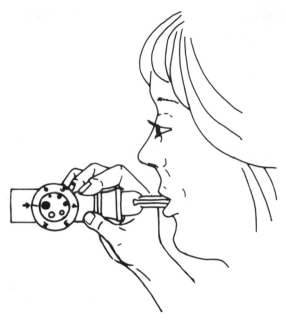

FIG. 4-38. *Inspiratory muscle training (Bell CW, Blodgett D, Goike CA et al: Home Care and Rehabilitation in Respiratory Medicine, p 46. Philadelphia, JB Lippincott, 1984)*

Therapeutic Objective

To improve respiratory muscle strength and endurance for pulmonary rehabilitation and the prevention or recurrence of respiratory failure.

Criteria for Termination

Undefined. This technique may require a continuous training program to prevent deconditioning effects when exercise is decreased. The training level of exercise may be higher than maintenance level. Discontinue patients who do not show peak inspiratory pressure improvement.

Contraindications

Uncooperative patients.

Procedure

For most situations resistive breathing offers ease of use, simplicity, and portability.

Strength training: Use a training program of multiple repetitions of short-duration exercise with rest between each period of exercise. Allow patient to set breathing rate. Change resistance orifice to progress patient.

Endurance training: Use a training program of low intensity and longer duration with no rest periods. Allow patient to set breathing rate. Change resistance orifice to progress patient.

Individualized exercise prescriptions are appropriate for respiratory muscle training just as they are for an overall exercise program.

Exact guidelines for this program of exercise have yet to be defined. Frequency, duration, intensity, schedules, mode of exercise as well as supervision have varied from study to study. As more information becomes available, appropriate parameters will be identified.[1]

Hazards

- Hypoxemia from increased oxygen consumption during exercise

Special Considerations

- Combine strength and endurance training when indicated.
- Supplemental oxygen during training sessions alleviates hypoxemia and improves exercise tolerance.
- Patients most likely to benefit from this technique include the COPD and neuromuscular patients.
- Allow patient to set breathing rate.
- Monitor tidal volume and breathing rate.

REFERENCE

1. Sobush D, Dunning M, McDonald K: Exercise prescription components for respiratory muscle training: Past, present, and future. Resp Care 30, No. 1: 34–42, 1985

BIBLIOGRAPHY

Bell W et al: Home Care and Rehabilitation in Respiratory Medicine, pp 45–47. JB Lippincott, Philadelphia, 1984

Belman M, Mittmau C: Ventilatory muscle training improves exercise capacity in chronic obstructive pulmonary disease patients. Am Rev Respir Dis 121:273–280, 1980

Buscaglia A, St Marie M: Oxygen saturation during chest physiotherapy for acute exacerbation of severe chronic obstructive pulmonary disease. Respir Care 28, No. 8:1009–1013, 1983

Cherneack R: Physical therapy. Am Rev Respir Dis (Suppl) 122, No. 5:25–27, 1980

Frownfeter D: Chest Physical Therapy and Pulmonary Rehabilitation. Chicago, Year Book Medical Pub, 1978

Gaskell DV, Webber BA: The Brompton Hospital Guide to Chest Physiotherapy, 4th ed. Boston, Blackwell Scientific Publications, 1980

Harris J, Bonita J: Indications and procedures for segmental bronchial drainage. Respir Care 20, No. 1:12, 1975

Hill J: Effects of chest physiotherapy on $TcPO_2$ values in neonates. Pulmonary Medicine and Technology 1, No. 10:27–29, 1984

Marini J: Postoperative atelectasis: Pathophysiology, clinical importance and principles of management. Respir Care 29:5, 516–528, 1984

Pardy R et al: New effects of inspiratory muscle training on exercise performance in chronic airflow limitation. Am Rev Respir Dis 123:421–425, 1981

Sobush D, Dunning M, McDonald K: Exercise prescription components for respiratory muscle training: Past, present and future. Resp Care 30, No. 1:34–42, 1985

Sonne L et al: Effect of inspiratory resistive training on muscle strength and endurance in severe chronic obstructive lung disease (abstr). Am Rev Resp Dis 123:63, 1981

Zack M, Palange A: Oxygen supplemented exercise of ventilatory and nonventilatory muscles in pulmonary rehabilitation. Chest 88, No. 5:669–675, 1985

5

airway management
Diane Blodgett
William DeForge

The purpose of airway management is to provide and maintain a clear and patent airway and protect the patient from aspiration. Airway management procedures include the insertion of artificial airways; or, the maintenance of those airways through suctioning, tracheal lavage, and humidification; and the use of cuff care techniques, tracheostomy care procedures, and other techniques which ensure that the objectives are met.

This chapter describes commonly used artificial airways and procedures for their insertion and use, and the care of tubes once they are in place. Tables giving characteristics of endotracheal and tracheostomy tubes are also provided.

These airway management techniques are common ones that all RT personnel should know and use. Of course, there are hazards involved with each technique just as there are benefits; these hazards are described under each individual procedure.

The criterion for termination of all these procedures is the return of the patient's ability to maintain a clear and patent airway.

OROPHARYNGEAL AIRWAY

Description

Curved device made out of plastic, rubber, or metal that is inserted into the oral cavity. This rigid or semirigid airway conforms to the shape of the pharynx and is positioned

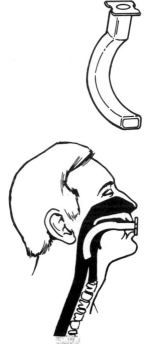

FIG. 5-1. *Oropharyngeal airway*

externally by a flange. Once in place the airway projects into the inferior oropharynx, providing a patent airway.

Therapeutic Objective

To maintain a patent airway, to facilitate the removal of secretions from the oropharynx, and to aid ventilation.

Criterion for Termination

Ability of patient to maintain a clear, patent, unobstructed airway.

Contraindications

Patients who do not regain a patent airway with this device.

Procedure

1. Hyperextend the neck.
2. Open the mouth either with a tongue depressor or a crossed thumb and index finger.
3. Insert the tip of the airway into the mouth. (The curve of the device should be at 180 degrees to the mouth curve.)
4. Gently rotate the airway upwards into position.
5. Position airway.
6. Clear oropharynx of secretions.
7. Tape airway into place.

Special Considerations

- Select the proper size from those listed below:

  00: Newborn

  0: Infant

  1: Child 1–3 years old

  2: Child 3–8 years old

  3: Large child–small adult

  4: Adult

  5: Large adult

  6: Large adult
- Tape the airway in place without totally occluding the mouth.
- Short-term use only.
- Many types are available; all have the same objective.

Hazards

- Gagging and aspiration
- Obstruction of airway if size of device is inappropriate
- Gastric insufflation if airway is too large
- Necrosis if airway is left in too long
- Occlusion of airway if mouth care is not provided

Maintenance

- Keep oral pharyngeal cavity free from pooling secretions.
- Change airway if occluded with secretions.

• Reposition airway frequently.
• Provide mouth care frequently.

NASOPHARYNGEAL AIRWAY

Description

Hollow, slightly curved device of flexible rubber or plastic that is inserted into the nasal cavity. Usually cone-shaped to prevent total passage into the nasopharynx.

Therapeutic Objective

To maintain a patent airway and to facilitate the removal of secretions from the nasopharynx.

Criterion for Termination

Ability of patient to maintain a patent, unobstructed airway.

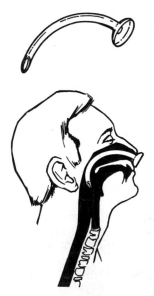

FIG. 5-2. *Nasopharyngeal airway*

Contraindications

Not for use in small children or patients with blocked nasal passages or nasal trauma.

Procedure

1. Lubricate the tip of the airway with water-soluble jelly.
2. Extend neck slightly.
3. Gently pass the tip of the airway through the external nares, aiming downward.
4. Position the tube.
5. Check for adequate air exchange.
6. Suction if necessary.
7. Secure the tube.

Special Considerations

- Select the proper size.
- If flange is not wide enough, insert large safety pin through the external end of the airway to prevent slippage.
- Short-term use only.
- Do not force the airway; if unable to pass device through one nostril, try the other.
- Useful for patients when oral cavity is not accessible.

Hazards

- Obstruction of airway with secretions
- Gastric insufflation with airway that is too large
- Necrosis of tissue if airway is left in place over extended period of time
- Airway that is too long can cause obstruction.

Maintenance

- If possible, reposition tube from one nostril to the other q8h.
- Keep airway free of secretions by providing adequate humidification and suctioning of secretions when necessary.
- Change airway if there is any question of obstruction.

ESOPHAGEAL OBTURATOR AIRWAY (EOA)

Description

Emergency device consisting of an occluded, cuffed tube that is passed into the esophagus (holes in the upper portion of the tube allow for air passage), a pilot balloon, a mask to cover the face and nose, and a 15 mm universal port to provide for support of ventilation by artificial means.

Therapeutic Objectives

To provide a patent airway, to prevent aspiration of gastric secretions, and to protect the airway.

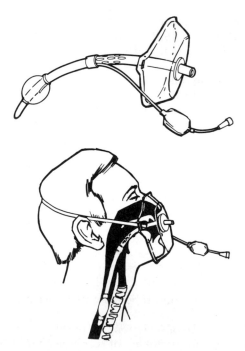

FIG. 5-3. *Esophageal obturator*

Criteria for Termination

Placement of endotracheal or tracheostomy tube; patient able to maintain patent airway; end of emergency situation.

Contraindications

Children, conscious patients, patients with damage to the esophagus (*e.g.*, that caused by ingestion of caustic material).

Procedure

1. Check integrity of the balloon by inflating with a syringe.
2. Lubricate the tip of the obturator with a water-soluble lubricant.
3. Attach mask and lock in place.
4. With the patient in the supine position, open patient's mouth and lift jaw with thumb and index finger without hyperextending the neck.
5. Insert the tube along the right side of the mouth through the pharynx and into the stomach.
6. Inflate the balloon with about 30 cc of air.
7. Attach manual resuscitator and begin ventilation, or ventilate by placing mouth on the adapter.
8. Auscultate chest to ensure proper placement.

Special Considerations

- Use only when endotracheal intubation is not possible.
- Do not use for severe face or head injuries.
- Breath sounds should be heard clearly when manual resuscitation provides a breath. No air should be heard entering the stomach. If air is heard entering the stomach, remove the EOA and reinsert.
- If patient starts to breath, remove mask.
- Have suction equipment at hand during extubation.
- Always deflate cuff before removal of tube.

Hazards

- Tracheal intubation
- Trauma to the esophagus or airway
- Gastric dilation with improper cuff inflation.
- Esophageal rupture during vomiting with EOA in place.

Maintenance

- Clean and decontaminate after each use.

ESOPHAGEAL GASTRIC TUBE AIRWAY

Description

A modification of the esophageal obturator airway, this cuffed device also has an opening for the insertion of a nasogastric tube to allow decompression of the stomach. There is a pilot balloon for cuff inflation. Ventilation takes place through a separate port in the mask.

Therapeutic Objective

To provide a patent airway, to prevent aspiration of gastric contents, and to allow decompression of the stomach with the insertion of a nasogastric tube.

Criteria for Termination

Placement of endotracheal or tracheostomy tube, patient able to maintain patent airway, end of emergency situation.

Contraindications

Children, conscious patients, patients with damage to the esophagus (*e.g.,* that caused by ingestion of caustic material).

Procedure

1. Check balloon integrity by inflating with a syringe.
2. Lubricate the tip of the tube with a water-soluble lubricant.

3. Clean any foreign materials from the airway.
4. With the patient supine, open mouth and lift jaw with thumb and index finger without hyperextending the neck.
5. Insert the airway along the right side of the mouth, through the pharynx, and into the stomach. Inflate the balloon.
6. After attaching a manual resuscitator or placing mouth on mask adapter, begin ventilation.
7. Auscultate chest to ensure proper placement.
8. Insert nasogastric tube to decompress the stomach.

Special Considerations

- Use when endotracheal intubation is impossible.
- Do not use for severe head and face injuries.
- Breath sounds should be heard clearly without air entering the stomach.
- Have suction equipment ready.
- Deflate cuff prior to removal.
- Do not use in conscious or semiconscious patients, children, or patients with esophageal damage.

Hazards

- Tracheal intubation
- Trauma to the airway or the esophagus
- Gastric dilation with inadequate cuff volumes

Maintenance

- Clean and decontaminate after use.

ENDOTRACHEAL TUBE

Description

An endotracheal tube is a long, hollow, slightly curved airway inserted either nasally or orally into the trachea. This tube, usually made of rubber or semirigid plastic, may or may not be cuffed. There is a standard 15 mm removable adapter for each size.

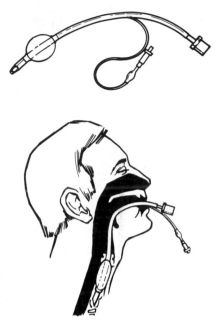

FIG. 5-4. *Oral endotracheal tube*

Therapeutic Objectives

To maintain a patent airway, to relieve airway obstruction, to prevent aspiration, to provide an effective means of maintaining tracheobronchial hygiene, and to facilitate mechanical ventilation.

Criteria for Termination

Ability of patient to maintain a patent airway and adequate spontaneous ventilation.

Contraindications

In extensive trauma to the head or total obstruction of upper airway, tracheostomy may be indicated instead of endotracheal intubation.

TABLE 5-1. GENERAL CHARACTERISTICS
OF ENDOTRACHEAL TUBES

Semirigid rubber or plastic tube

Curved to conform to anatomical position

Standard 15 mm universal adapter

May be uncuffed or cuffed

Radiopaque tip

Length markers

Stylet may be used for insertion

Beveled end

Usually single-patient use

Procedure

INSERTION (OROTRACHEAL INTUBATION)

1. Place the patient in the supine position, with the neck hyperextended and the head slightly elevated above the shoulders.
2. Have the following equipment ready:
   a. Suction equipment.
   b. Various sizes of endotracheal tubes with adapters attached.

TABLE 5-2. CHARACTERISTICS OF ENDOTRACHEAL TUBES
(BY AGE)

ADULT	*PEDIATRIC*
Cuff Type I	
High residual volume	Uncuffed or cuffed
Low-pressure cuff	Sizes 2.5–5.0 mm
Floppy	May have tapered end (Cole)
Less chance of pressure damage to trachea	May have T configuration for use with circle ventilator setup
Cuff Type II	
Low residual volume	
High-pressure cuff	
Should only be used with minimal-leak technique	
Sizes 5.0–10 mm	

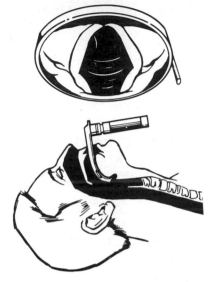

FIG. 5-5.   *Endotracheal intubation*

    c. Laryngoscope with straight or curved blades, sizes 1–4.
    d. Syringe to inflate cuff.
3. Select the appropriate tube size.
4. If tube has a cuff, test the cuff for proper inflation.
5. Select the blade and attach to the laryngoscope handle.
6. Insert the blade into the right side of the mouth and move the tongue to the left.
7. Lift up slightly as the blade is moved forward.
8. Visualize the epiglottis and arytenoid cartilages.
9. Suction to clear secretions in the airway.
10. Insert the endotracheal tube along the right side of mouth.
11. While visualizing the cords, direct the tube through the opening of the glottis.
12. Advance the tube past the glottis so the top of the cuff is through the opening.
13. Remove the blade.
14. Inflate the cuff of the tube until a minimal or no-leak condition is met.

15. Inflate the lungs with a manual resuscitator to check for tube placement. (Bilateral, equal breath sounds should be heard.) If air is heard entering the stomach, remove the tube at once and reinsert after proper ventilation and reoxygenation.
16. Obtain chest x-ray film to verify proper position.

INSERTION (NASOTRACHEAL INTUBATION)

1. Place the patient in the supine position with the neck hyperextended and the head slightly above the shoulders.
2. Have the following equipment ready:
   a. Suction equipment.
   b. Various sizes of endotracheal tubes with adapters attached.
   c. Laryngoscope with straight or curved blades, sizes 1–4.
   d. Syringe to inflate cuff.
   e. Magill forceps.

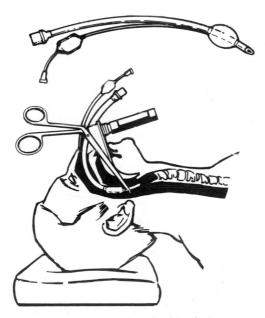

FIG. 5-6. *Nasal tracheal intubation*

3. Select the appropriate size tube.
4. If tube has a cuff, test the cuff for proper inflation.
5. Select the blade and attach to the laryngoscope handle.
6. Choose the larger of the nares for tube passage.
7. Anesthetize nostril with a lidocaine spray; also spray nostril with an alpha-adrenergic agent to prevent bleeding.
8. Lubricate tip of tube with a viscous lidocaine jelly.
9. Insert tube into nostril pointing backward and downward. Advance tube slowly.
10. Do not force tube if resistance is met.
11. After the tube is in the hypopharynx, visualize the cords with the laryngoscope.
12. Clear secretions with suction.
13. Grasp tube with Magill forceps and pass tube through the vocal cords, advancing until the balloon is past the level of the cords.
14. Remove blade and forceps.
15. Inflate the cuff.
16. Attach manual resuscitator.
17. Auscultate the chest to ensure bilateral breath sounds.
18. If air is heard entering the stomach, remove the tube at once and reinsert after proper ventilation and reoxygenation.
19. Secure tube with tape.
20. Obtain chest x-ray to verify proper placement.

INSERTION (BLIND NASOTRACHEAL INTUBATION)

Used when actual visualization of the vocal cords is not possible.

1. Place the patient in the supine position with the neck hyperextended and the head slightly above the shoulders.
2. Have the following equipment ready:
   a. Suction equipment.
   b. Various sizes of endotracheal tubes with adapters attached.
   c. Laryngoscope with straight or curved blades, sizes 1–4.
   d. Syringe to inflate cuff.
   e. Magill forceps.
3. Select the appropriate size tube.

4. If tube has a cuff, test the cuff for proper inflation.
5. Select the blade and attach to the laryngoscope handle.
6. Choose the larger of the nares for tube passage.
7. Anesthetize nostril with a lidocaine spray; also spray nostril with an alpha-adrenergic agent to prevent bleeding.
8. Lubricate tip of tube with a viscous lidocaine jelly.
9. Insert tube into nostril pointing backward and downward. Advance tube slowly.
10. Do not force tube if resistance is met.
11. With the tube in the pharynx, listen for breath sounds by placing ear next to the end of the tube.
12. Advance the tube through the vocal cords on inhalation; extrusion of the tongue may aid with this maneuver.
13. Attach manual resuscitator.
14. Auscultate the chest to ensure bilateral breath sounds.
15. If air is heard entering the stomach, remove the tube at once and reinsert after proper ventilation and reoxygenation.
16. Secure tube with tape.
17. Obtain chest x-ray to verify proper placement.

EXTUBATION

1. Approach the patient and explain the procedure.
2. Have equipment at hand to reintubate the patient if necessary.
3. Suction the airway to clear secretions.
4. Suction the upper airway to clear secretions.
5. Deflate the cuff.
6. Instruct the patient to take a deep breath and cough.
7. As the patient coughs, pull the tube gently but smoothly from the patient's airway.
8. Suction mouth if necessary.
9. Watch for signs of obstruction.
10. If stridor is present, racemic epinephrine can be given by nebulizer.

Special Considerations

- Lubricate the tube by applying water-soluble lubricant to the cuff area. With nasal intubations, use lidocaine jelly

and be sure to anesthetize the nostril and nasopharynx.
- Do not attempt to pass tube if the glottis is closed.
- Do not inflate cuff just by "feeling" the resistance against the syringe or the pressure in the pilot balloon.
- Monitor cuff pressure (see Chap. 7).
- Use sterile technique when suctioning patient.
- If bilateral equal breath sounds are not heard, the tube may
    a. Be in the esophagus (if no breath sounds are heard). Remove tube and reinsert. (Capnographs have been used to verify tube placement. Carbon dioxide monitors will indicate no exhaled CO_2 when esophagus is intubated.)
    b. Be in the right mainstem bronchus (if sounds are only heard on right). If tube is in the right mainstem bronchus, pull back on tube slightly and again listen for breath sounds.
- Take x-ray to check the placement of the tube.
- Mark a line on the endo tube so that if the tube does move it can easily be moved back to the correct position.
- Curved blade is placed into the vallecula, above the epiglottis.
- Straight blade is placed beyond the epiglottis.
- Keep intubation equipment close by to reintubate the patient if accidental extubation occurs.
- Move tube to different positions in the mouth to prevent necrosis.
- Extrusion of the tongue may aid with intubation via the nasal route.

Hazards

- Misplacement of tube into esophagus or right mainstem bronchus
- Traumatic intubation: Chipping of teeth, bleeding, tissue damage to airway, rupture of trachea, damage to nasal passage, sinusitis, epistaxis
- Loss of communication route
- Infection
- Hypoxia
- Bradycardia

- Glottic and subglottic edema
- Vocal cord paralysis or ulceration
- Obstruction of airway by placement of the distal tube orifice against the airway
- Normal humidification mechanisms bypassed
- Tracheomalacia with long-term intubation and high cuff pressures

Maintenance

- Keep airway patent by adequately humidifying the inspired air and suctioning secretions when necessary.
- Monitor cuff pressures.
- Change the placement of tube from one side of mouth to the other.
- Change bite block and tape or tie that holds tube in place.

DOUBLE LUMEN ENDOBRONCHIAL TUBE

Description

A double lumen endobronchial tube is a long, hollow, curved airway with two separate tubes combined in one, two separate cuffs, and two standard 15 mm adapters for each lumen.

Therapeutic Objectives

To allow independent ventilation of each lung, to allow independent positive end-expiratory pressure (PEEP) or continuous positive airway pressure (CPAP) to each lung, to provide a means for independent bronchial hygiene, and to facilitate better ventilation in certain disease processes.

Criteria for Termination

Improvement in underlying disease process, end of postoperative period.

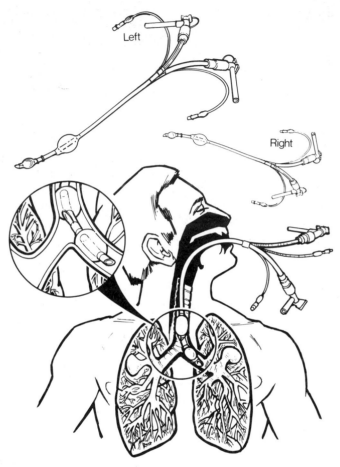

FIG. 5-7. *Endobronchial tube for selective lung ventilation*

Contraindications

Use when independent lung ventilation is necessary.

Procedure

1. Place patient in the supine position with the neck hyperextended and the head slightly above the shoulders.

2. Have the following equipment ready: suction equipment, endobronchial tube, laryngoscope with straight or curved blades, syringe to inflate cuffs.
3. Test both cuffs for proper inflation.
4. Insert blade into right side of the mouth.
5. Lift slightly as blade is advanced forward.
6. Clear secretions if needed.
7. Visualize epiglottis and arytenoid cartilage.
8. Insert endobronchial tube through the cords and advance well beyond the cords.
9. Inflate cuffs and ventilate each lumen, ensuring that breath sounds are heard on each side.
10. Obtain chest x-ray to ensure proper placement.

Special Considerations

- Lubricate tube to facilitate ease of placement.
- Do not attempt to pass tube if epiglottis is closed.
- Monitor cuff pressures.
- Use sterile technique when suctioning the patient.
- X-ray must be obtained to ensure proper placement.
- If breath sounds are not heard on the left, the balloon may be obstructing the left mainstem bronchus and the tube may have to be repositioned.
- The end of the tube should be in the right mainstem bronchus.
- Do not use with documented left mainstem obstruction.

Hazards

- Obstruction of the left mainstem
- Hazards inherent with endotracheal intubation (chipped teeth, tissue damage, etc.)
- Trauma to the carina
- Difficulty with insertion
- Loss of communication route
- Infection
- Intubation of the esophagus
- Hypoxemia
- Cardiac arrythmias
- Not intended for long-term ventilation
- Elimination of the normal body humidification system

Maintenance

• Keep airway patent by providing adequate humidity and suctioning the airways when necessary.
• Monitor cuff pressure (see Chap. 7).

TRACHEOSTOMY TUBE

Description

A trach tube, a hollow, curved airway inserted into the tracheostomy site, may or may not be cuffed. The tubes can be made of metal, nylon, Silastic, Teflon, or other synthetic material. Most have an inner and an outer cannula with an obturator for insertion.

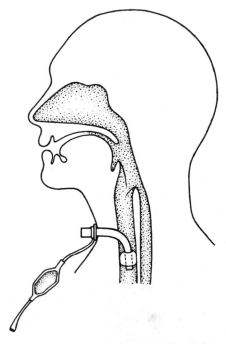

FIG. 5-8. *Cuffed tracheostomy tube (Bell CW, Blodgett D, Goike CA et al: Home Care and Rehabilitation in Respiratory Medicine, p 224. Philadelphia, JB Lippincott, 1984)*

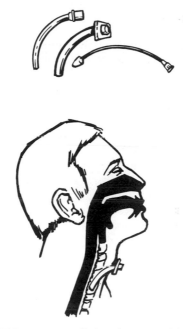

FIG. 5-9. *Uncuffed tracheostomy tube*

Therapeutic Objective

To maintain an airway that bypasses an upper airway obstruction, to facilitate long-term mechanical ventilation, to provide an effective means of maintaining tracheobronchial hygiene, and (with a cuffed tube) to prevent aspiration.

Criteria for Termination

Coughing mechanism intact, underlying disease under control, patient able to maintain patent airway.

Contraindications

None.

Procedure

CLEANING THE INNER CANNULA (FOR TWO-CANNULA TRACHEOSTOMY TUBES)

1. Approach the patient and explain the procedure.
2. Assemble the necessary equipment:
   a. Trach care tray: Either disposable or hospital-prepared
   b. Solutions: 2% to 3% hydrogen peroxide, sterile distilled water, sterile normal saline
   c. Suction equipment
   d. Scissors
   e. Sterile 4 × 4s
3. Place patient in semi–Fowler's position.
4. Wash hands with a germicidal soap.
5. Prepare the tracheostomy care equipment:
   a. Open sterile drape and position on work surface.
   b. Open sterile 4 × 4s onto drape.
   c. Fill two basins: one with sterile water, one with hydrogen peroxide.

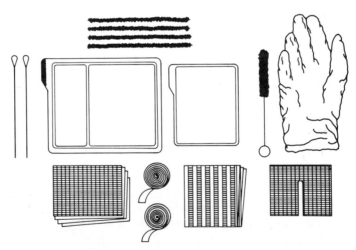

FIG. 5-10. *Tracheostomy care: Cleaning (Bell CW, Blodgett D, Goike CA et al: Home Care and Rehabilitation in Respiratory Medicine, p 235, Philadelphia, JB Lippincott, 1984)*

6. Prepare suction equipment.
7. Hyperoxygenate the patient.
8. Suction inner cannula if necessary.
9. Release lock of tracheostomy tube and remove inner cannula; place in basin of hydrogen peroxide.
10. Put on sterile gloves.
11. Clean inner cannula using cleaning brushes and pipe cleaners to remove mucus and crusts. Clean thoroughly.
12. Place inner cannula in basin of water.
13. Clean flanges of outer cannula with moistened cotton swabs. Use sterile 4 × 4s to wipe away secretions that patient may expectorate.
14. Use sterile wipes to dry inner cannula.
15. Place cannula on drape.
16. Suction outer cannula if necessary.
17. Gently reinsert inner cannula and lock in place.
18. Dispose of equipment.
19. A second inner cannula may be necessary if the patient cannot tolerate being deconnected from the ventilator.

CHANGING TRACHEOSTOMY TUBE BIB

1. Remove and discard soiled bib.
2. Cleanse around the tracheostomy tube with 4 × 4s moistened with a sterile solution of water or normal saline.
3. Dry area.
4. Replace new bib gently to prevent dislodgment of tube.
5. Dispose of equipment.

CHANGING TRACHEOSTOMY TUBE TIES

1. Prepare clean ties: Fold one end of each tie over 1" inch and cut a slot ¼" to ⅓" long.
2. Remove one soiled tie.
3. Insert uncut end through hole in side of flange of the outer cannula and thread this end through the slit on the other end; pull through until secure.
4. Repeat for second tie.
5. Secure a knot with the ties. For patient comfort, tie knot on side of neck. You should be able to insert two fingers between the tie and the patient's neck.

CHANGING THE TRACHEOSTOMY TUBE

1. Approach the patient and explain the procedure. Hyperoxygenate the patient.
2. Gather necessary equipment; Suction equipment, gloves, 4 × 4s, new tube.
3. Suction the patient through the trach tube and then suction the oropharynx. Deflate cuff and have the patient cough (or inflate the lungs).
4. Again, hyperoxygenate the patient.
5. Prepare the tube for insertion (*i.e.,* cuff checked, ties attached, obturator in place).
6. Put on sterile gloves.
7. Remove the trach bib and cut the trach ties carefully.
8. As the tube is being removed, have the patient exhale forcefully or cough.
9. Remove secretions from opening with sterile 4 × 4s.
10. Quickly, but gently, insert new tracheostomy tube into stoma, aiming back and downward.
11. Remove obturator and insert inner cannula if necessary.
12. Secure tube in place.
13. Hyperoxygenate the patient.
14. Suction the airway if necessary.

REMOVING THE TRACHEOSTOMY TUBE

Note: You can prepare the patient by progressing to smaller tubes.

1. Approach the patient and explain the procedure.
2. Assemble the necessary equipment: Suction equipment, sterile 4 × 4s, tape, gloves.
3. Place patient in semi-Fowler's position.
4. Wash hands.
5. Suction patient through the trach tube and then suction oropharynx. Deflate cuff.
6. Put on gloves and have 4 × 4s open and ready.
7. Cut the trach ties.
8. Have the patient cough as the trach is being removed.
9. Clear the stoma of any secretions with a 4 × 4.
10. Cover the stoma with a 4 × 4 and tape into place.
11. Check the patient's respirations and ability to clear the

airway (have patient place fingers over gauze covering stoma and cough). Monitor vital signs and watch for signs of obstruction.

12. Dispose of equipment.

Special Considerations

- Change trach dressing when moist.
- Do not use dressing when drainage from fresh trach has diminished.
- Always keep a second trach tube at the bedside.
- Tape the obturator to the head of the bed.
- Do not use tracheostomy tubes with detachable cuffs since they present a great hazard to the patient.
- Choose the trach tube that meets the needs of the patient (Tables 5-3, 5-4, 5-5).
- X-ray should be taken after the initial tracheostomy is done and the tube has been inserted. This will check the placement of the tube.
- Fenestrated tubes facilitate preparation for extubation.

TABLE 5-3. GENERAL CHARACTERISTICS OF ADULT TRACH TUBES

- Curved or angled shape to facilitate insertion and removal.
- Obturator with blunted end to facilitate insertion of outer cannula.
- Cuffed tube used to prevent aspiration, to permit mechanical ventilation, to position cannula in center of trachea. Cuff (inflatable balloon on distal end of trach cannula) seals upper airway from lower airway.
- Uncuffed tube used to maintain tracheostomy over long period of time when there is no danger of aspiration or need for mechanical ventilation.

Adult Tube Size Conversion

FRENCH SIZE	METRIC SIZE ID	JACKSON SIZE
24	5.5	4
27	6.0–6.5	5
30	7.0	6
33	7.5–8.5	7
36	8.5	8
39	9.0–9.5	9
42	10.0	10

TABLE 5-4. GENERAL CHARACTERISTICS OF PEDIATRIC
TRACH TUBES

• Anatomically shaped
• Usually no inner cannula
• No cuff. Cuff would occupy too much space.
• Correct size must be chosen to prevent necrosis or leaks.
• Obturator may or may not be available.

Pediatric Tube Size Conversion

METRIC SIZE ID	JACKSON SIZE	FRENCH SIZE
2.5	00	13
3.0	0	15
3.5	1	16.5
4.0	2	18
4.5–5.0	3	21
5.5	4	24
6.0–6.5	5	27

Hazards

SURGICAL

• Bleeding
• Aspiration of blood
• Subcutaneous/mediastinal emphysema
• Pneumothorax
• Cardiopulmonary arrest

POSTOPERATIVE SURGICAL

• Postoperative hemorrhage
• Infection
• Airway obstruction
• Tube displacement
• Blockage of tube

LATE COMPLICATIONS

• Tracheal stenosis (narrowing)
• TE fistula–innominate artery hemorrhage
• Tracheomalacia (loss of cartilaginous support)
• Tracheal erosion
• Herniation of cuff

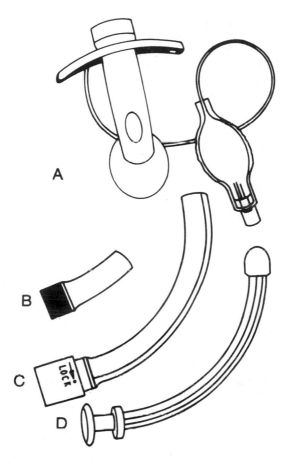

FIG. 5-11. *Fenestrated tracheostomy tube with cuff. (A) Fenestrated trach tube, (B) plug, (C) inner cannula, (D) obturator (Bell CW, Blodgett D, Goike CA: Home Care and Rehabilitation in Respiratory Medicine, p 226. Philadelphia, JB Lippincott, 1984)*

- Infection; sepsis
- Displacement of tube
- Subcutaneous emphysema
- Hemorrhage
- Difficulty clearing secretions spontaneously
- Loss of communication route

(*Text continues on p. 176.*)

TABLE 5-5. TYPES AND CHARACTERISTICS OF TRACH TUBES

NAME	MATERIAL	CUFF	INNER CANNULA	OBTURATOR	SIZES	DISPOSABLE	SPECIAL CONSIDERATIONS
Adult Tubes							
Jackson trach tube	Silver Stainless steel	No (can be attached, but not recommended)	Yes	Yes	3–10 mm metal	No	Come in sets that do not always have interchangeable parts. Lock keeps inner cannula in place. Trach care should be given PRN
Air-lon trach tube	Nylon	No (can be attached, but not recommended)	Yes	Yes	3–8 mm nylon	No	Come in sets that do not always have interchangeable parts. Trach care should be given PRN
Martin laryngectomy tube	Silver Stainless steel Nylon	No	Yes	Yes	8 mm and 10 mm	No	Come in sets that do not always have interchangeable parts. Lock keeps inner cannula in place. Trach care

should be given PRN. Tube larger and shorter than trach tube. Tube usually placed higher in neck

Portex blue line trach tube	Siliconized plastic (PVC) impregnated with silicone	Yes (low-pressure) / Some without cuff	Yes (with some models)	Yes	French: 24–39 (6–10 mm)	Yes	Impregnated—no crusting on inside and outside of tube. 15 mm standard connection. One-way valve to inflate pilot balloon/monitor pressure. Double-cuffed tube available. Extra-length tube available. Radiopaque blue line makes tube easy to identify on x-ray
Mallincrodt	Plastic (PVC) impregnated with silicone	Yes (low-pressure)	Yes (with some types)	Yes	5–10 mm	Yes	Standardized connector; one-way inflation valve

(Continued)

TABLE 5-5. TYPES AND CHARACTERISTICS OF TRACH TUBES (Continued)

NAME	MATERIAL	CUFF	INNER CANNULA	OBTURATOR	SIZES	DISPOSABLE	SPECIAL CONSIDERATIONS
Shiley PRV–LPC	PVC	Yes (low-pressure)	Yes; some disposable	Yes	French: 26–39 (5–9 mm); 4, 6, 8, 10	Yes	During cuff inflation, any pressure above 25 mm Hg in cuffs is vented to atmosphere. Once relief valve is closed, cuff pressure can increase as patient or tube changes position. Trach care should be given PRN. Radiopaque
Dow Corning Silastic	Silicone rubber	Some with and some without cuffs	Yes	Yes	Some with 0–9; some without	Yes	Radiopaque. Trach care should be given PRN for those tubes with inner cannula
Bivona Fome-Cuf Tube	Silicone and polyurethane	Yes (low-pressure)	No	Yes	#5–#9	Yes	Coating on tube prevents crusting of secretions and blocking of airway.

								Comments
								15 mm standard connection. Radiopaque tip for ease of location on X-ray. To insert tube, air is first withdrawn from cuff; tube is then inserted and cuff is allowed to inflate when port is opened to atmosphere. Do not use Trach Talk with this type of tube (the airway will be completely occluded!)

Pediatric Tubes

Portex infants trach tube	Transparent PVC	No	No	No	No	3.1–6.0 mm	Yes	Not always radiopaque. Small lumen—keep clear of secretions. Shape of flange and tube designed and adapted to anatomy of newborn or small infant

(Continued)

173

TABLE 5-5. TYPES AND CHARACTERISTICS OF TRACH TUBES (Continued)

NAME	MATERIAL	CUFF	INNER CANNULA	OBTURATOR	SIZES	DISPOSABLE	SPECIAL CONSIDERATIONS
Shiley pediatric trach tube	PVC	No	No	Yes	00–3 (3.1–4.8 mm)	Yes	15 mm standard connector. Radiopaque. Ninety-degree distal end, cut to minimize the possibility of blocking against anterior wall. Anatomically shaped flange and cannula for pediatric use. Small lumen—keep clear of secretions
Rusch flexible trach tube	PVC with stainless steel spiral	No	No	Intubating tube	3–6 mm	Yes	Standard 15 mm connector. Fully flexible tube that adapts to any change in position

							Comments
							of trachea. Adjustable flange with lock ring that prevents movement when tube is in place. Spiral—radiopaque. Small lumen size—keep clear of secretions. Intubating guide is also suction catheter
Jackson trach tube	Silver Stainless steel	No	Yes	Yes	No	OD–3 (3.1–4.8 mm) No	Comes in sets that do not always have interchangeable parts. Lock keeps inner cannula in place. Small lumen—keep clear of secretions. Trach care should be given PRN

- Natural humidification mechanisms are bypassed
- Pneumothorax

Maintenance

- Keep airway patent by adequately humidifying the inspired air and suctioning secretions when necessary.
- For tubes with an inner cannula, trach care should be given q2–q4 hours the first 24 hours, q8h and PRN thereafter.
- Change bib and ties when soiled.
- Change tube once a week or more often when indicated (*i.e.,* cuff blown).
- Monitor cuff pressures (see Chap. 7).

TRACHEOSTOMY BUTTON

Description

A short, straight, hollow plastic tube inserted into the tracheostomy stoma. This device does not occlude the airway and allows unobstructed airflow between the upper and lower airways.

Objective

To maintain a tracheostomy stoma.

Criterion for Termination

Ability of patient to maintain patent airway.

Contraindications

Patients who aspirate.

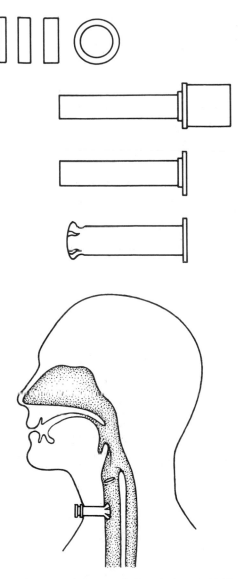

FIG. 5-12. *Tracheostomy button (Bell CW, Blodgett D, Goike CA et al: Home Care and Rehabilitation in Respiratory Medicine, p 229. Philadelphia, JB Lippincott, 1984)*

Procedure

DETERMINING THE SIZE

1. Select a trach button the same size (external diameter) as the patient's tracheostomy.
2. Measure length of stoma. Insert a marked curette into the stoma and measure from the anterior wall of the trachea to the skin surface.
3. Place spacers on trach button to adjust length of cannula.

INSERTION OF TRACH BUTTON

1. Approach the patient and explain the procedure.
2. Lubricate the button with a water-soluble jelly.
3. Gently insert the button into the stoma.
4. Insert closure plug into button.
5. Check for proper placement and fit (should be firm and secure).

REMOVAL OF TRACH BUTTON

1. Approach the patient and explain the procedure.
2. Remove the closure plug.
3. Gently pull the cannula straight out.

Special Considerations

- Keep stoma site clean and dry.
- Make sure appropriate size button is inserted.
- Adapter available with 15 mm fitting to use with various respiratory therapy treatment modalities.
- Make sure button is sterile before using.
- French sizes 27–42.

Hazards

- Infection
- Localized irritation

Maintenance

- Remove and clean button twice a week with hydrogen peroxide and sterile water.

TRACH TALK

Description

Device attached to tracheostomy tube which allows the patient to talk.

Objective

To allow a patient with a tracheostomy tube in place to speak without placing his finger over the tube opening.

Procedure

1. Approach the patient and explain the procedure and device.
2. Deflate the cuff for patients with a cuffed tracheostomy tube.

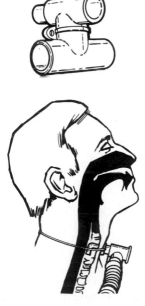

FIG. 5-13. *Trach talk*

3. Check the patency of the upper airway by having the patient occlude the opening to the trach.
4. Ask the patient to speak.
5. If the patient can speak, attach the trach talk to the tube via the standard 15 mm adapter or fit the tube with an adapter.
6. For continuous aerosol therapy, large-bore tubing can be attached to either inlet.

Special Considerations

- Suction the patient through port or by removal of trach talk.
- Aerosol therapy can be administered concurrently with the use of this device.
- Do not use this device with a tight-fitting trach tube or a trach tube with cuff inflated, or with a patient who has an airway obstruction above the tracheostomy tube.
- Fits most standard trach tube fittings.
- Check the patient frequently during initial trial for signs of increased work of breathing or obstruction.

Hazards

- Occlusion of airway
- Increased work of breathing

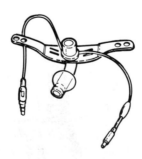

FIG. 5-14. *Trach talk tube*

Maintenance

- Disposable device that can be disassembled for decontamination.
- Keep valve clear of secretions to prevent sticking.

NASAL OR ORAL PHARYNGEAL SUCTIONING

Description

Nasal pharyngeal suctioning is the removal of secretions from the lower and upper airway through a suction catheter that is placed proximal to the secretions. This catheter is positioned directly into the pharynx or trachea via the nasal or oral cavity.

Objectives

To maintain a patent airway; to remove secretions from those patients who are unable to do so themselves.

Criteria for Termination

Ability of patient to expectorate on his own; elimination of underlying disease causing increase in sputum production.

Contraindication

None; see Hazards.

Procedure

1. Approach the patient and explain the procedure.
2. Obtain necessary equipment (suction source, regulator bottle, connecting tubing, sterile suction catheter, sterile gloves, sterile saline or water, sterile basin, water-soluble jelly).

3. Wash hands.
4. Hyperoxygenate the patient by increasing the FiO_2 and position the patient (usually in semi-Fowler's).
5. Using aseptic technique, fill basin with sterile water or saline.
6. Open catheter and glove(s).
7. Turn on regulator and adjust suction source to appropriate vacuum.
8. Put on glove(s) and attach catheter to connecting tubing.
9. Lubricate catheter with jelly.
10. Insert catheter through the nares along the base of the nasal cavity (or through oral cavity).
11. Have the patient breathe slowly with his mouth open.
12. As the patient inhales, advance the catheter, twisting it slightly.
13. When the patient coughs as you advance the catheter, you have reached the trachea.
14. Place thumb over the control port of the catheter and apply suction.
15. Release thumb and withdraw catheter slightly.
16. Again apply suction and release.
17. Withdraw catheter, suction, release suction in this order until catheter is removed.
18. Clear catheter and tubing with sterile solution.
19. Reoxygenate the patient and suction against if necessary.
20. Extrusion of the tongue may aid with entry into the trachea.
21. Dispose of equipment.

Special Considerations

- Disposable suction kits may contain any or all of these sterile items: Gloves, catheter, water, basin.
- Do not suction for more than 15 to 20 seconds.
- Always preoxygenate or hyperinflate the patient before suctioning.
- Use the appropriate size of catheter (see Table 5-6).
- Suction catheters should never be reused.
- Coude (curved-tip) catheter may facilitate the removal of secretions from the right mainstem bronchus.

TABLE 5-6. CATHETER SIZES AND VACUUM SETTINGS FOR ORAL/NASAL SUCTIONING

AGE OF PATIENT	SUCTION CATHETER SIZE (FRENCH)	VACUUM SETTINGS	
		Portable	Wall
Infants	5	3–5 in Hg	60–100 torr
Children	6–12	5–10 in Hg	100–120 torr
Adults	12–16	7–15 in Hg	120–150 torr

- Turn patient's head to left to facilitate suctioning of right bronchus.
- Turn patient's head to right to facilitate suctioning of left bronchus.

Hazards

- Hypoxia.
- Cardiac arrythmias.
- Bradycardia.
- Airway mucosal trauma.
- Infection.
- Atelectasis.
- Apnea.

Maintenance

- Dispose of equipment after each use.

TRACHEOBRONCHIAL SUCTIONING

Description

Tracheobronchial suctioning removes secretions from the lower airway through a catheter placed proximal to the secretions. This procedure is accomplished directly through an endotracheal, tracheostomy, or laryngectomy tube.

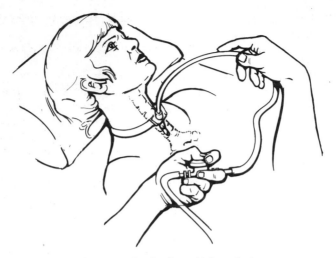

FIG. 5-15. *Tracheobronchial suctioning*

Criteria for Termination

Removal of endotracheal or tracheostomy tube; ability of patient to maintain a patent unobstructed airway.

Contraindications

None; see Hazards.

Procedure

1. Approach the patient and explain the procedure.
2. Obtain necessary equipment (suction source, regulator bottle, connecting tubing, sterile suction catheter, sterile gloves, sterile saline or water, sterile basin).
3. Wash hands.
4. Hyperoxygenate the patient by increasing the FiO_2 or sighing the patient.
5. Position patient (usually semi-Fowler's).
6. Using aseptic technique, fill basin with sterile saline or water.

7. Turn on regulator and adjust suction source to appropriate vacuum setting.
8. Put on glove(s) and attach catheter to connecting tubing.
9. Remove oxygen–administering device.
10. Pass catheter through opening of endotracheal or tracheostomy tube without applying suction.
11. When resistance is met a cough should be elicited. Withdraw the catheter slightly and apply suction. Place thumb over the control port of the catheter and apply suction.
12. Release thumb and withdraw catheter slightly.
13. Again apply suction and release.
14. Withdraw catheter, suction, release suction in this order until catheter is removed.
15. Clear catheter and tubing with sterile solution.
16. Hyperoxygenate patient and suction again if necessary.

Special Considerations

- Disposable suction kits may contain any or all of these sterile items: Gloves, catheters, water basin.
- Do not suction for more than 15 to 20 seconds.
- Always hyperoxygenate and hyperinflate the patient before suctioning.
- Use appropriate size catheter (see Table 5-6).
- Always use sterile technique.
- Suction catheters should never be reused.
- Coude (curved-tip) catheter may facilitate the removal of secretions from the right mainstem bronchus.
- Keeping the patient's head in the midline position appears to be the most reliable practice when attempting to remove secretions from the left mainstem bronchus.
- To loosen secretions, 3 to 5 ml of sterile saline can be instilled into the endotracheal, tracheostomy, or laryngectomy tubes before suctioning.
- Give artificially ventilated patient 2 to 3 hyperinflation breaths via the respirator following the instillation and preceding the suction procedure.
- For the patient who is not being ventilated, give 2 to 3 hyperinflation breaths by manual resuscitator with oxy-

gen following the instillation and preceding the suction procedures.

Hazards

- Hypoxia
- Cardiac arrythmia
- Atelectasis
- Bradycardia
- Infection
- Airway mucosal trauma
- Apnea

Maintenance

- Dispose of equipment after each use.

MINIMAL-LEAK TECHNIQUE

Description

This technique allows a small amount of air to escape from the lower airway to the upper airway around the inflated cuff of an endotracheal or tracheostomy tube.

Objective

To inflate the cuff of an endotracheal or tracheostomy tube to the point where a small amount of air is allowed to

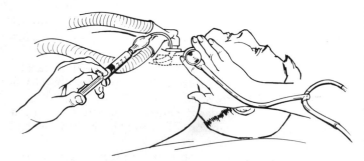

FIG. 5-16. *Minimal-leak technique*

escape around it. This technique minimizes the chances of tracheal wall damage from an overinflated cuff.

Criteria for Termination

Removal of tube or the necessity of using a no-leak technique.

Contraindications

Patients who are in danger of aspirating.

Procedure

1. Approach the patient and explain the procedure.
2. Place a stethoscope diaphragm on the patient's trachea.
3. Start to inject air into the inflating tube which is connected to the endotracheal or tracheostomy tube cuff.
4. Cycle the ventilator and inject air into the inflating tube (or have the spontaneously breathing patient take a deep breath).
5. At the end of inspiration, listen over the trachea for a small air leak.
6. If no leak is heard, repeat the procedure while slightly deflating the cuff.
7. Check pressure in cuff (see Chap. 7).

Special Considerations

- Can only be used on patients using PEEP or CPAP when ventilators are adjusted to compensate for the leak.
- Important to choose correct tube size.
- For all patients, ventilator settings must be adjusted to compensate for leak.

Hazards

- Aspiration around cuff
- Hypoventilation

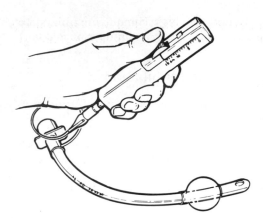

FIG. 5-17. *Cuff check*

Maintenance

• Check leak routinely.
• If there is no apparent airflow around cuff or if air leak is large, repeat procedure.
• Check cuff volume and pressure routinely when patient is repositioned and when cuff is reinflated.

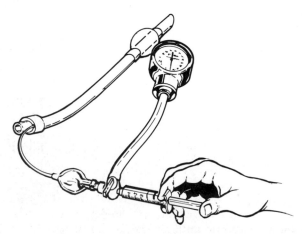

FIG. 5-18. *Cuff pressure measurement*

• Do not exceed pressures of 25 mm Hg, which is considered the upper safety limit for cuff pressure.

NO-LEAK TECHNIQUE

Description

During the no-leak technique, the cuff is inflated to totally block the passage of air between the upper and lower airway. No air is allowed to pass around the endotracheal or tracheostomy tube when the cuff is inflated.

Therapeutic Objective

To totally occlude the space between the tracheal wall and the cuff on a cuffed endotracheal or tracheostomy tube; to prevent air from leaking around the cuff.

Criterion for Termination

When total occlusion is no longer necessary, switch to minimal-leak technique.

Contraindication

Patient who can tolerate a small leak in the ventilator patient interface (minimal leak preferred).

Procedure

1. Approach the patient and explain the procedure.
2. Place a stethoscope diaphragm on the patient's trachea.
3. Start to inject air into the inflating tube which is connected to the endotracheal or tracheostomy tube cuff.
4. Cycle the ventilator and inject air into the inflating tube.
5. At the end of inspiration, listen over the trachea for a small leak. No air movement should be heard.
6. Repeat procedure until air leak is eliminated.
7. Check pressure in cuff (see Chap. 7).

Special Considerations

- Use technique only where cuff pressures and volumes are carefully monitored.
- May be indicated for patients on PEEP or CPAP, patients who aspirate, and patients with decreased lung compliance.

Hazards

- Erosion of the tracheal wall due to high cuff pressures
- Mucosal damage
- Tracheal dilation

Maintenance

- Check cuff volume and pressure routinely when repositioning patient and reinflating cuff.
- Do not exceed cuff pressures of 25 mm Hg.

SPUTUM INDUCTION

Description

The patient is given a heated aerosol or ultrasonically nebulized acetylcysteine or hypertonic saline to induce a productive cough. A sterile specimen is then collected.

Therapeutic Objectives

To assist the patient in raising sputum; to collect a sputum sample for examination.

Procedure

1. Approach the patient and explain the procedure.
2. Administer aerosol therapy (hypertonic saline, etc.) for 20 to 30 minutes.
3. After about 10 minutes encourage the patient to cough.
4. If the patient can raise any sputum, have him expectorate into a sterile specimen container.

5. Label specimen and send to laboratory immediately.
6. Continue aerosol therapy up to 30 minutes to induce a productive cough.

Special Considerations

- Wear mask and gown when collecting specimen from contagious patient.
- Collect specimen in a sterile cup.
- Do not use bacteriostatic agent in aerosolized solution.
- Label specimen with name, date, time, and source of specimen.

Hazards

- Possible spreading of contagious disease
- Bronchospasm

Maintenance

- Label and send specimen to laboratory immediately.
- See aerosol therapy treatment procedure.

SPECIMEN TRAP

Description

This device traps secretions in a sterile specimen container during a suctioning procedure.

Therapeutic Objective

To collect, by suctioning, a sterile specimen for examination.

Procedure

1. Assemble suction equipment.
2. Place trap in line with suction catheter and suction tubing.

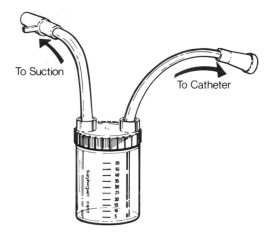

FIG. 5-19. *Specimen trap*

3. Turn on and adjust suction control.
4. Suction the patient using an aseptic technique.
5. Collect specimen in the vial.
6. After sample is obtained, remove suction catheter and tubing from trap.
7. Seal trap by connecting the two open parts.
8. Label trap and send specimen to laboratory immediately.

Special Considerations

• Some traps may have suction catheter attached, necessitating the replacement of catheter cap with a plain cap.
• If secretions are thick, rinse catheter clear with a small amount of saline.
• Label specimen with name, date, time, and source of specimen.

Hazards

• Spread of infection
• Hazards associated with suctioning procedure (bradycardia, hypoxia)

Maintenance

• Dispose of all materials after use.
• Send specimen to laboratory immediately.

BIBLIOGRAPHY

Adams AL, Cane RD, Shapiro BA: Tongue extrusion as an aid to blind nasal intubation. Crit Care Med 10, No. 5: 335–336, 1982

Baker PO, Baker JP, Koen PA: Endotracheal suction techniques in hypoxemic patients. Resp Care 28, No. 1563–1568, 1983

Burton G, Hodgkin JE (eds): Respiratory Care: A Guide to Clinical Practice. Philadelphia, JB Lippincott, 1984

Demers RR: Complications of endotracheal suctioning procedures. Resp Care 27 No. 4: 453–457, 1982

Ellis PD, Billings DM: Cardiopulmonary Resuscitation: Procedures for Basic and Advanced Life Support. St Louis, CV Mosby, 1980

Fluck J, Owen R: Use of an apnea monitor to verify endotracheal intubation. Resp Care 30, No. 11: 974–976, 1985

Fluck RR, Wagner IJ, Wiezalis CP: Letter: Proper insertion of the esophageal obturator airway. Resp Care 28, No. 12: 1604–1606, 1983

Ishida T, Yoshia I, Morita Y, Shirae K: Quantitative analysis of tracheal damage. Crit Care Med 11, No. 4: 283–285, 1983

Kruser K: Letter: Preoxygenation and hyperinflation associated with suctioning. Resp Care 27, No. 10; 1286, 1982

Kubota Y, Magaribuchi T et al: Selective bronchial suctioning in the adult using a curve-tip catheter with a guide mark. Crit Care Med 10, No. 11: 767–769, 1982

Kvetan V, Carlon G, Howland W: Acute pulmonary failure in asymmetric lung disease: Approach to management. Crit Care Med 10, No. 2: 114–118, 1982

McPherson SP: Respiratory Therapy Equipment, 3rd ed. St Louis, CV Mosby, 1984

Off D, Braun SR, Tompkins B, Bush G: Efficacy of the minimal leak technique in cuff inflation in maintaining proper intracuff pressures for patients with cuffed artificial airways. Resp Care 28, No. 9: 1115–1120, 1983

Powner DJ, Eross B, Grenvik A: Differential lung ventilation with PEEP in the treatment of unilateral pneumonia. Crit Care Med 5, No. 4: 170–172, 1977

Rindfleisch S, Tyler M: Duration of suctioning: An important variable. Resp Care 28, No. 4: 457–459, 1983

Shinnick JP, Freedman AP: Bronchoscopic placement of a double-lumen endotracheal tube. Crit Care Med 10, No. 8: 544–545, 1982

Stauffer JL, Silvestri RC: Complications of endotracheal intubation, tracheostomy, and artificial airways. Resp Care 27, No. 4: 417–435, 1982

6

assisted mechanical ventilation

William DeForge
Contribution by
Richard Branson

The respiratory care practitioner who plays an important role in the care of the critically ill patient must have a complete and thorough understanding of the indications, contraindications, hazards, and weaning techniques associated with critically ill patients supported by mechanical ventilators. The respiratory care practitioner must also have a thorough understanding of the operation of the equipment.

In general, mechanical ventilation is indicated in patients with alveolar hypoventilation or shunt hypoxia in which a ventilation/perfusion mismatch exists. In both cases the patient cannot provide adequate ventilation for oxygen delivery to the cells and carbon dioxide removal. Thus, ventilation supplied by mechanical means must be adequate to achieve both. In attaining this goal, the respiratory care practitioner must use technical, pathological and physiological knowledge in the critical care clinical situation.

Table 6-1 describes the general guidelines for providing ventilatory support in adults. These general guidelines do not apply to patients with chronic hypoxia and with chronic carbon dioxide retention. With these patients the therapist should evaluate the blood pH, PaO_2 levels, and the patient's clinical appearance. In these patients a falling pH (below 7.35) usually indicates impending respiratory failure.

TABLE 6-1. GUIDELINES FOR VENTILATORY SUPPORT IN ADULTS

DATA	NORMAL RANGE	TRACHEAL INTUBATION AND VENTILATION INDICATED
Mechanics		
Respiratory rate	12–20	>35
Vital capacity (ml/kg of body weight)	65–75	<15
FEV$_1$ (ml/kg of body weight)	50–60	<10
Inspiratory force (cm H$_2$O)	75–100	<25
Oxygenation		
PaO$_2$ (mm Hg)	75–100 (air)	<70 (on mask high concentration O$_2$)
P(A–aD)O$_2$ (mm Hg)	25–65	>450
Ventilation		
PaCO$_2$ (mm Hg)	35–45	>55
V̇D/V̇T	0.25–0.40	>0.60

(Pontoppidan H et al: Acute Respiratory Failure in the Adult, p 60. Boston, Little, Brown & Co, 1973)

CLASSIFICATION OF VENTILATORS

One of the most confusing areas of respiratory care is ventilator classification, which describes the mechanism of operation of the ventilator. However, all ventilators, regardless of their classification, must complete the following four basic phases:

1. Inspiratory phase
2. The transition from inspiration to exhalation
3. Exhalation phase
4. Transition from exhalation to inspiratory phase

TABLE 6-2. PHASES OF A VENTILATOR

PHASE I	PHASE II	PHASE III	PHASE IV
Inspiratory phase (generating force)	Inspiratory/ expiratory phase (cycling mechanism)	Expiratory phase (retard, PEEP, NEEP, ZEEP)	Expiratory/ inspiratory phase (mode of ventilation)

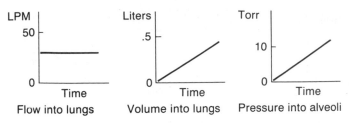

FIG. 6-1. *Characteristics of constant-flow generators (After Burton G, Hodgkin JE: Respiratory Care: A Guide to Clinical Practice, 2nd ed, p 559. Philadelphia, JB Lippincott, 1984)*

Positive-pressure ventilators are of four types:

1. Constant-flow generators
2. Nonconstant-flow generators
3. Constant-pressure generators
4. Nonconstant-pressure generators

Constant-flow generators provide a constant, non-changing, flow rate regardless of compliance change in the circuit or the patient.

A nonconstant-flow generator provides a consistent breath-to-breath flow characteristic but the inspiratory flow rate varies throughout the inspiratory phase. This mimics normal breathing.

Constant-pressure generators maintain the same pressure from breath to breath, but as the pressure in the circuit rises the flow rate falls until the preset pressure is reached.

A nonconstant-pressure generator has pressure changes;

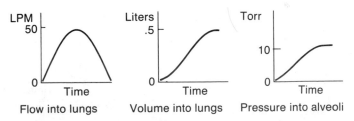

FIG. 6-2. *Characteristics of nonconstant-flow generators (After Burton G, Hodgkin JE: Respiratory Care: A Guide to Clinical Practice, 2nd ed, p 560. Philadelphia, JB Lippincott, 1984)*

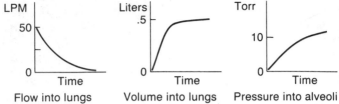

FIG. 6-3. *Characteristics of constant-pressure generators (After Burton G, Hodgkin JE: Respiratory Care: A Guide to Clinical Practice, 2nd ed, p 560. Philadelphia, JB Lippincott, 1984)*

however, the pressure pattern remains the same from breath to breath without regard to changes in compliance.

During Phase II of the ventilator cycle, inspiration changes to expiration. Four variables allow inspiration to end and expiration to begin: time, pressure, volume, or flow. These are cycling mechanisms and each has its own specific indications. Table 6–3 lists the most common ventilators and their classification.

Time–cycled ventilators terminate gas flow in the patient circuit when a preselected time interval has been reached. The volume of gas delivered can be determined by the formula Vol = Flow (vol/time) × (time). Changes in patient compliance or airway resistance alter the actual amount of volume delivered. The volume and pressure vary when a preset inspiratory pressure relief level is reached prior to the end of the inspiratory cycle time, when the remaining volume will be vented. When the preset time interval is reached before the preset pressure relief,

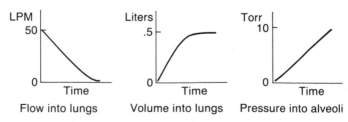

FIG. 6-4. *Characteristics of nonconstant-pressure generators (After Burton G, Hodgkin JE: Respiratory Care: A Guide to Clinical Practice, 2nd ed, p 651. Philadelphia, JB Lippincott, 1984)*

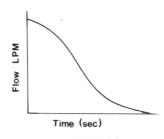

FIG. 6-5. *Pressure generator-inspired flow*

then the actual volume delivered will be higher. Keep this in mind when using this type of ventilation mode for patients with high airway resistance or low compliance.

Pressure-cycled ventilators change from inspiration to expiration when the ventilator attains a preset pressure level. It is easy to see why the volume delivered can be so variable when this type of ventilation is used. Patients with high airway resistance or low compliance receive less delivered tidal volume since the preset pressure limit will be reached sooner. The inspiratory flow rate set on the machine alters the actual amount of delivered tidal volume. A high inspiratory flow rate causes an increase in turbulence as well as peak airway pressure. This allows the preset pressure limit to be reached sooner, resulting in smaller delivered tidal volume.

Volume-cycled ventilators end inspiration when a preset volume has been attained. The volume of gas actually received by the patient varies with patient compliance, airway resistance, and the type of ventilator circuit. Generally, tubing compliance accounts for 2.5 to 5.0 cc/cm H_2O volume loss. For example, with a volume set for 1000 cc, the peak airway pressure at 30 cm H_2O, and with tubing

(*Text continues on p. 202.*)

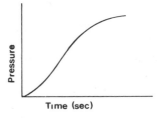

FIG. 6-6. *Pressure generator-inspired obstruction*

TABLE 6-3. CLASSIFICATION OF SPECIFIC VENTILATORS

| | | PHASE I | | | PHASE II | | | | PHASE III | | | | | | PHASE IV | | |
Ventilator	MMV	Pressure Support	Constant-Flow Generator	Non-constant-Flow Generator	Pressure Generator	Inspiratory Plateau	Time-Cycled	Pressure-Cycled	Volume-Cycled	ZEEP	PEEP	Expiratory Retard	Assistor	Controller	Assistor/Controller	IMV	SIMV
Bennett MA-1					X				X	X	X	X	X	X	X		
Bennett MA-2				X	X	X			X	X	X		X	X	X	X	X
Bennett 7200		X			X	X	X	X	X	X	X			X	X		X
Gill 1					X	X			X	X	X		X	X	X	X	
Bourns Bear 1			X		X				X	X	X		X	X	X	X	X
Bear 2			X	X		X	X		X	X	X			X	X		X
Bear 5		X	X	X	X	X	X		X	X	X			X	X	X	X
Foregger 210			X				X			X	X		X	X	X	X	
Ohio 560					X	X			X				X	X	X		
Ohio CCV					X	X					X		X	X	X	X	

Ventilator	1	2	3	4	5	6	7	8	9	10	11
Searle VVA		X	X	X	X		X		X		
Monaghan 225		X	X	X	X		X		X		
Emerson 3PV				X			X	X		X	X
Emerson IMV		X	X	X			X	X			X
Emerson 3MV		X	X	X			X	X			X
Veriflo CV 2000		X	X	X	X		X				
Veriflo 200	X		X	X	X		X				
Engstrom ECS 2000			X	X		X					X
Engstrom ER 300		X	X	X			X	X	X		X
Engstrom Erica		X	X	X			X	X	X		X
Siemens 900B		X	X	X	X	X	X	X	X	X	X
Siemens 900C			X	X	X	X	X	X	X		X
Biomed 10-5		X	X	X	X		X	X	X	X	X
Hamilton		X	X	X			X	X	X	X	X
Ohmeda CPU-1		X	X	X			X	X	X	X	X

(1)
$$P = \frac{n8L\ \dot{V}}{\pi\ r^4}$$

(2)   constant
$$\uparrow P \cong \frac{\dot{V}}{r^4 \downarrow}$$

(3)
$$P \cong \frac{\dot{V}\downarrow}{r^4 \downarrow}$$

P = Pressure

n = Viscosity

L = Length

$\dot{V}$ = Flow (ml./sec.)

π = Constant

r^4 = Tube radius

FIG. 6-7. *(1) Poiseuille's Law. (2) All the constants are removed from Poiseuille's Law and r^4 (radius of airway) decreases, thus increasing airway resistance when $\dot{V}$ remains constant as with constant flow generators. The P (back pressure) is increased, resulting in less volume passing by the obstructed area. (3) Pressure generator phenomenon, where r^4 decreases, $\dot{V}$ also decreases, thus diminishing the degree of back pressure and resulting in better ventilation past the obstruction.*

compliance factor of 3 cc/cm H_2O, the actual volume delivered is 910 cc (1000 − [30 × 3] = 910). The volume of 90 cc remains in the circuit. This volume distends the tubing. Even though a monitoring spirometer may indicate that the volume returned equals the volume set on the machine, the patient doesn't necessarily receive that volume. This factor becomes very important when ventilating patients with respiratory distress syndrome and high peak airway pressures. Very high peak pressures and low compliance can result in considerable loss of volume. If the peak pressure is changed to 50 cm H_2O, the delivered volume falls to 850 cc. In spite of this characteristic drawback, the volume ventilator remains the most popular ventilator on the market.

Flow-cycled ventilators end inspiration when the gas flow falls below a preset level independent of inspiratory time, tidal volume, or airway pressure. A classic example of this type of ventilator is the Bennett PR-2.

Phase III of the ventilatory cycle, the exhalation phase, is

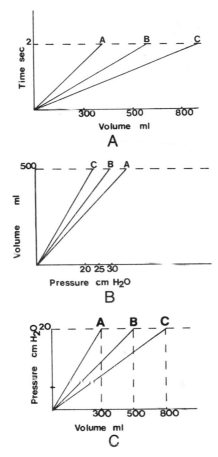

FIG. 6-8. *Delivery volume and pressure changes that occur in lung when using (A) time-cycled machines, (B) volume-cycled machines, and (C) pressure-cycled machines. (A) ↓ compliance or ↑ airway resistance. (B) Normal compliance and airway resistance. (C) ↑ compliance or ↓ airway resistance.*

normally a passive maneuver, allowing equilibration of pressure between the lungs and the atmosphere. This is termed *ZEEP*, or zero end-expiratory pressure. Sometimes during exhalation an expiratory retard is used to prevent early closure of the airways, especially in COPD. This method mimics pursed-lip breathing.

Another method, PEEP, has been widely used in the treatment of hypoxemia unresponsive to large tidal volumes and a high F_IO_2. *PEEP*, or positive end-expiratory pressure, maintains a certain level of pressure in the patient circuit at all times. PEEP improves oxygenation and decreases intrapulmonary shunt by increasing functional residual capacity. This is done by recruiting unventilated alveoli and by expanding already open alveoli. Unfortunately, PEEP has also been associated with some adverse effects which must be considered within the total clinical picture before PEEP is instituted. Since PEEP is widely used, respiratory care practitioners should be familiar with all aspects of this treatment modality. Table 6-4 lists the benefits and adverse effects of PEEP.

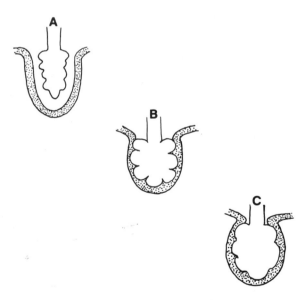

FIG. 6-9. *Three stages of alveoli with PEEP application*

A. Collapsed	B. Normal	C. Overdistention
↓ FRC	FRC	↑ FRC
↓ Compliance	Compliance	↓ Compliance
↑ Closing vol.	Closing vol.	↓ Closing vol.
↑ % shunt	% shunt	↓ % shunt
↑ PVR	PVR	↑ PVR
↓ V̇/Q̇	V̇/Q̇ = 0.8	↑ V̇/Q̇

TABLE 6-4. POSSIBLE BENEFITS AND ADVERSE EFFECTS OF PEEP

POSSIBLE BENEFITS	POSSIBLE ADVERSE EFFECTS
Increases FRC	Barotrauma
Decreases closing volume	Pneumothorax
Increases oxygenation	Pneumomediastinum
Redistributes lung water, decreasing alveolar edema	Subcutaneous emphysema
	Decreased compliance
	Decreased venous return
	Decreased cardiac output
	Increased PVR
	Decreased PaO_2 with high levels of PEEP
	Increased intracranial pressure

Going from a collapsed alveolus to a normal expanded alveolus improves the FRC, compliance, closing volume, and % shunt without increasing PVR. This is considered *best PEEP* or the best compliance level. If no deleterious effects occur with these parameters, the level of PEEP can usually be increased by 2 cm to 5 cm H_2O. If PaO_2 or cardiac output falls with an increase in the PVR, then the PEEP level is too great and should be decreased.

Sometimes the best compliance level will not result in the best PaO_2, or even in a sufficient PaO_2 level. In these cases, the shunt is so bad (usually above 15%) that it takes a higher level of PEEP to reduce it, even though the compliance will decrease and PVR will increase when the best compliance level is exceeded. The increased PVR results in a drop in cardiac output (CO), but with fluid therapy and vasopressors CO can be maintained. Thus, the % shunt will be reduced and O_2 transport can be maintained. This application of PEEP is known as *optimal PEEP*.

Some of the common abbreviations utilized in Phase III are NEEP, ZEEP, and PEEP. NEEP = negative end-expiratory pressure; ZEEP = zero end-expiratory pressure; PEEP = positive end-expiratory pressure.

The last phase of the ventilator cycle is the change from exhalation to inhalation. This phase is designated by the

(*Text continues on p. 208.*)

TABLE 6-5. CAPABILITIES OF VENTILATORS

	TIDAL VOL. (ML)	RATE (MIN)	INSPIRATORY HOLD (SEC)	EXPIRATORY RETARD	PEEP (CM H₂O)	PRESSURE LIMIT (CM H₂O)	INSPIRATORY FLOW RATE (BPM)	F₁O₂ RANGE (%)
Bennett MA-1	100–2200	6–60	NA	NA	0–20	10–80	15–100	21–100
Bennett MA-2	100–2200	0–60	0–2	NA	0–45	20–80	0–125	21–100
Bennett 7200	100–2500	5–70	0–2	NA	0–45	10–120	10–180	21–100
Gill 1	150–2100	6–60	0–2	NA	0–50	20–100	10–120	21–100
Foregger 210	80–8000	0.5–75	0.2–2	NA	0–35	20–110	12–120	21–100
Ohio 560	100–2000	6–60	0–2	NA	0–12	10–100	180	21–100
Ohio CCV	100–2000	5–40	0–2	NA	0–15	10–100	240	21–100
Searle VVA	300–2200	5–60	0–3	NA	0–20	10–100	20–200	21–100
Monaghan 225	100–3300	4–60	NA	NA	0–20	10–100	10–100	21–100
Emerson 3PV	20–2200	5–99	NA	NA	0–25	10–100	1.2–260	21–100
Emerson IMV	200–2200	0.2–22	NA	NA	0–25	50–100	5.5–60	21–100
Emerson 3MV	0–2000	0–26	NA	NA	0–50	0–120	0–180	21–100
Veriflo CV 2000	10–2000	8–60	NA	NA	0–20	20–100	12–100	21–100

Engstrom ECS 2000	20–1600	6–60		NA	0–20	10–100	0.2–384	21–100
Engstrom Erica	100–2000	4–40	% of insp. time	NA	0–30	0–120	0.2–90	21–100
Engstrom ER 300	20–2200	12–35	0–0.8	NA	0–20	30–90	1–264	21–100
Bear 1	100–2000	0.5–60	0–2	NA	0–30	0–100	20–120	21–100
Bear 2	100–2000	0.5–60	0–2.0	NA	0–50	0–120	10–120	21–100
Bear 5	50–2000	0–150	0–2.0	NA	0–50	0–50	5–150	21–100
Siemens 900B	5–30 l (MV)*	6–60	% of insp. time	NA	optional	10–100	variable	21–100
Siemens 900C	0.5–40 l (MV)	5–120	% of insp. time	NA	0–50	20–120	variable	21–100
Biomed 10-5	0.5–3000	5–150	% of insp. time	NA	0–35	0–120	5–120	21–100
Hamilson	20–2000	.5–60	% of insp. time	NA	0–50	0–110	0–180	21–100
Ohmeda CPU-1	60–6000	.5–66	% of insp. time	NA	0–30	0–100	0–120	21–100

* MV = minute ventilation

mechanism that triggers the machine to deliver a tidal breath (mode of ventilation). If the patient initiates inspiration, then it is termed *assist*. This means that each time the patient "assists," a breath will be delivered by the machine. Usually a preset rate is set to deliver a certain number of breaths per minute should the patient fall below that rate or become apneic. This mode is termed *assist/control*. If the patient cannot control the number of breaths delivered, the mode is termed *control*.

Another mode of ventilation, *IMV*, or intermittent mandatory ventilation, has a preset machine rate, but the patient can breathe between the machine breaths at his own tidal volume. The breaths between the machine breaths will not be pressurized breaths. Some ventilators are equipped to synchronize the machine breaths with the patient's inspiratory effort. Advantages of *SIMV,* or synchronized intermittent mandatory ventilation, include the following:

1. Reduces mean intrathoracic pressure.
2. Enhances the "thoracic pump."
3. Allows patient to regulate own $PaCO_2$ level.
4. Reduces incidence of barotrauma.
5. Allows muscles of inspiration and exhalation to be utilized and coordinated.
6. Easier to wean patient from mechanically assisted ventilation.

Modes of ventilation used vary from hospital to hospital, region to region, and even doctor to doctor. This text will not discuss or compare benefits and adverse effects of the various modes of ventilation. See the Bibliography for additional resource information.

Once the four phases every ventilator must pass through for a complete ventilatory cycle of inspiration and exhalation are understood, it becomes easier to place ventilators within this classification system (Table 6–3). Table 6–5 lists the same ventilators with some of their capabilities. Understanding these capabilities aids in the proper selection of a ventilator for specific therapeutic needs, such as PEEP, inspiratory plateau, large or small tidal volumes, or pressure support.

With an understanding of the classification system and the various capabilities of specific ventilators, the respiratory clinician can make an educated selection of a ventilator for clinical use. The clinician should be able to select a ventilator that can accomplish the therapeutic needs outlined in a physician's order including

1. Mode of ventilation (*i.e.,* assist, control, assist/control, IMV, or SIMV)
2. Tidal volume (usually between 10 ml–15 ml/kg of body weight)
3. Respiratory rate (usually between 10–15 breaths per minute)
4. Inspiratory/expiratory ratio (usually 1/2)
5. Desired FiO_2
6. Sigh volume ($1.5–2 \times \dot{V}T$)
7. Sign frequency (at least every 5 minutes)
8. PEEP level, inspiratory plateau, or expiratory resistance if desired
9. Pressure support if necessary

Anticipate that some of the initial settings will need readjusting dependent upon each patient's response to the ventilator. Use normal arterial blood gas levels (*p*H 7.35–7.45, PaO_2 35–45) as the guidelines for any ventilator adjustments.

With a physician's order secured, the respiratory clinician can begin the procedure which will result in the connection of the ventilator to the patient's artificial airway.

CONNECTING VENTILATOR TO PATIENT

Description

Mechanical ventilation artificially supports patient ventilation by providing volume, gas flow, and concentration at a rate that is physiologically sound.

Therapeutic Objectives

• To maintain physiologic ventilation.
• To manipulate ventilatory pattern and airway pressure.
• To decrease work of breathing.

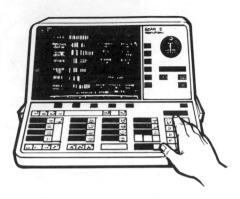

FIG. 6-10. *Bear 5 ventilator*

Criteria for Termination

See Weaning Criteria.

Contraindications

None; see Hazards.

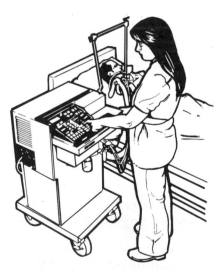

FIG. 6-11. *Puritan-Bennett 7200*

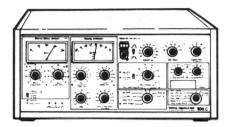

FIG. 6-12. *Servo 900C*

Procedure

1. Secure physician's order for MAV.
2. Select appropriate ventilator.
3. Connect ventilator to various power sources (*e.g.,* electrical outlet, O_2 system). Turn on.
4. Adjust sensitivity for mode of ventilation (*e.g.,* assist, control, assist–control, IMV, SIMV).
5. Adjust V_T (10 ml–15 ml/kg).
6. Adjust frequency to regulate $PaCO_2$ as desired.
7. Adjust desired FiO_2.
8. Adjust inspiratory flow as necessary to achieve the desired I/E ratio.
9. Adjust sigh volume and frequency to 1.5–2 × $\dot{V}_I$ every 4–12 minutes if sigh is prescribed.
10. Adjust pressure limits.
11. Using a test lung, manually cycle ventilator to ensure that it is functioning properly.
12. Connect ventilator circuit to patient's artificial airway.
13. Listen to patient's breath sounds and watch for chest excursion when ventilator cycles into inspiratory phase.
14. Adjust low and high pressure alarms.
15. Attach any additional monitoring devices and set the alarm limits (mass spectrometer, disconnect alarm, etc.).
16. After 20 minutes obtain arterial blood gas sample.
17. Adjust V_T or rate for desired pH and $PaCO_2$, and FiO_2 for desired PaO_2.

Special Considerations

- The patient on continuous ventilation needs a good humidifying system. Keep humidifier filled with sterile distilled water at all times.
- Monitor FiO_2 and inspired temperature on a continuous basis.
- Incorporate alarm systems that will alert you to high and low airway pressures and tidal volumes, power failure, inadequate delivered volumes.
- Never leave ventilator patient unattended for any length of time.
- Monitor the patient's physiologic data frequently to avoid complications (see Hazards).
- Obtain ABGs when changing ventilation parameters or with a changing clinical picture. Use oximetry or transcutaneous monitors to assist in physiological evaluation.

Hazards

- Airway:
  a. Occlusion and obstruction of airway
  b. Migration of tube into the right mainstem bronchus
  c. High cuff pressure leading to tracheal erosion
  d. Inadequate cuff pressures leading to a leak and volume loss
- Cardiovascular:
  a. Hypotension with increased intrathoracic pressures
  b. Decreased venous return
  c. Decreased cardiac output
  d. Decreased renal blood flow
  e. Decreased tissue oxygenation
- Decrease in cerebral blood flow
- Increase in intracranial pressure
- Atelectasis may occur if you use low tidal volumes without sigh:
  a. Decreased FRC
  b. Decreased compliance
  c. Increased closing volume
  d. Ventilation/perfusion mismatch
  e. Decrease in PaO_2
- Increased incidence of nosocomial infections

- Barotrauma:
  - a. Pneumothorax
  - b. Pneumomediastinum
  - c. Subcutaneous emphysema
- Pulmonary:
  - a. Increased dead space
  - b. Increased pulmonary vascular resistance
  - c. Increased intrapulmonary shunt
- Improperly trained or incompetent persons can be disastrous. All personnel involved with the ventilator should have a thorough understanding of the operation, beneficial effects, adverse effects, corrective measures, and trouble-shooting techniques for each type of ventilator.
- Equipment failure. This can be easily controlled by a competent respiratory clinician. The common complications associated with equipment failure are outlined below.

Common Equipment Failure

A. Circuit:
   1. Disconnect between ventilator and patient
   2. Obstruction from kink or water in the tubing
   3. Holes or tears in the tubing leading to leaks in the system
B. Ventilator:
   1. Electrical failure
   2. Source gas failure
   3. Altered ventilator settings
C. Humidification device:
   1. Decreased water supply
   2. Inappropriate temperature
   3. Leaks
D. Monitoring devices:
   1. Not activated
   2. Improper adjustment
   3. Malfunction

As stated previously, the respiratory clinician should be able to identify any of these complications.

Maintenance

• Change all tubing and humidifiers (patient circuit) daily.
• If tubing fills with condensate, empty water from circuit (not back into system).
• Change permanent filters following manufacturer's instructions.

HIGH FREQUENCY JET VENTILATION

High frequency jet ventilation is a new mode of ventilation recently approved by the FDA for treatment of bronchopleural and tracheoesophageal fistulas, and for diagnostic bronchoscopy. Use of HFJV for anything other than this requires a special permit from the FDA.

HFJV volume is delivered to the patient via short bursts of gas from a high-pressure gas source through a small injector cannula. Respiratory rates of up to 600/min have been used with this type of ventilation.

The volume delivered to the patient varies with several factors. When an electrical or pneumatic valve opens, gas flow begins accelerating in the cannula. The lateral pressure begins to drop to subatmospheric while gas entrainment surrounding the injector cannula takes place.

The amount of gas entrained depends upon velocity of jet gas flow, size of the jet cannula, size of the entrainment

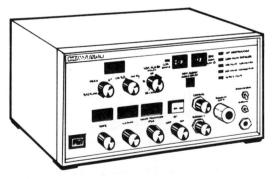

FIG. 6-13. *HFJV (jet ventilator)*

port, time of jet flow, and resistance distal to the jet flow. Changes in any of these result in changes in the delivered volume. For example, if an increase in jet flow velocity causes a greater drop in lateral pressure, the amount entrained will be larger. If the resistance distal to the jet injector increases for whatever reason, there will be less entrained gas and the volume delivered will be lower.

Basically, HFJV is controlled ventilation. The respiratory rate is controlled by the rate set on the machine. Although the patient cannot cycle the machine, he may breathe spontaneously at any time. One interesting finding is that after a patient has been on the jet ventilator for a few seconds, spontaneous respirations cease. This appears to be a reflexogenic response and occurs even at normal ventilation. At rates greater than 100/min, there is less suppression of respirations. Spontaneous respirations return 10 to 15 seconds after HFJV is discontinued.

HFJV also results in auto-PEEP. This auto-PEEP results from gas trapping that increases alveolar pressure without affecting proximal airway pressure. This auto-PEEP occurs when high driving pressures and high inspiratory times are used.

During conventional ventilation gas transport occurs via bulk flow and simple molecular diffusion. The delivered tidal volume is greater than the patient's physiologic dead space. With HFJV the tidal volume delivered is less than the physiologic dead space and therefore the mechanism of gas transport is different. When tidal volume is greater than dead-space volume, gas flows according to pressure gradients and follows the general laws of gas physics. With HFJV there is no pressure gradient. Flow probably occurs via turbulence, increased regional gas currents, increased mixing due to airway movements, vibration of gases in the airways, and convective flow.

Humidification of inspired gases during HFJV is very important. Humidifying the entrained gases alone, however, is not enough; the jetted gas must also be humidified. Generally 0.9% normal sterile saline is used for humidification of the jetted gasses. The two methods commonly used utilize Bernouilli's principle, along with an infusion pump, to ensure adequate humidity. The usual starting point is 10 cc to 15 cc/hr of normal saline/sterile water

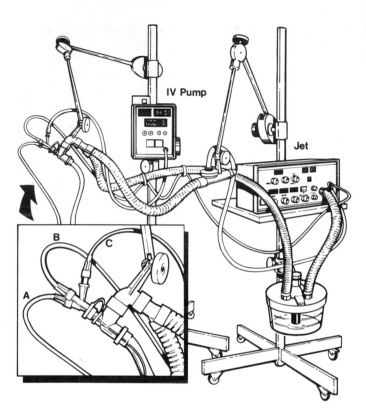

FIG. 6-14. *HFJV connection. (**A,** pressure monitoring line; **B,** jet injector port; **C,** humidity infusion line)*

infused directly into the jet line or entrained through another catheter juxtaposed to the jet injector cannula.

CONNECTING THE PATIENT TO THE HFJV

Description

HFJV supports the patient's ventilation in the face of airway disruption such as bronchopleural and tracheoesophageal fistulas. Volume is provided by a solenoid-controlled, high-pressure gas source forced through a narrow cannula.

Gas surrounding the injector cannula is entrained to add to the volume delivered.

Therapeutic Objectives

- To maintain adequate ventilation in the face of a physiologic air leak.
- To maintain ventilation at decreased peak airway pressures.

Criteria for Termination

Resolution of underlying problem.

Contraindications

Treatment of disease states other than bronchopleural or tracheoesophageal fistulas, or diagnostic bronchoscopies. (Special FDA permit needed for all other investigational purposes.)

Procedure

1. Secure physician order for HFJV.
2. Obtain informed consent from patient or someone authorized to sign.
3. Connect ventilator to appropriate power sources (electrical, gas, etc).
4. Adjust rate to 100, percent inspiratory time fraction to 33%, and drive pressure to 25 PSIG.
5. Begin with FiO_2 at 100 and decrease as tolerated.
6. Attach humidity line with infusion pump and ensure proper function. Set rate at 10 cc/hr; increase if necessary.
7. Connect ventilator to patient airway.
8. Closely monitor HR, BP, O_2 saturation via ear oximeter, and transcutaneous CO_2 and O_2 levels. Mass spectrometry has not been shown to be accurate in HFJV.
9. Adjust high and low pressure alarms.
10. Sample ABGs frequently until the patient stabilizes.
11. Titrate $PaCO_2$ to desired level by adjusting drive pressure. Increase drive pressure to decrease the $PaCO_2$; lower drive pressure to increase the $PaCO_2$ level.

12. Titrate PaO_2 to desired levels by adjusting the FiO_2 and inspiratory time fraction.

Special Considerations

- Monitor patient's vital signs and ventilatory status closely.
- Humidify entrained as well as jetted gases.
- Never leave patient on HFJV alone.
- Have conventional ventilator ready should the HFJV not be of benefit to the patient.
- Obtain ABG with any ventilator change.
- Increase % inspiratory time if increasing the drive pressure fails to produce desired carbon dioxide level.
- Turn off jet stream before suctioning the patient to prevent spread of infection.
- Bronchodilators may be entrained into system when needed.

Hazards

- Drying of airways with inadequate humidity
- Swelling of airways and mucosa with too much humidity.
- High peak airway pressures can be reached within 10 seconds with obstruction of exhalation outflow tract.
- Inadequate ventilation in patients with poor compliance.
- Do not use anesthetic gas with HFJV.

Maintenance

- Change tubing and humidifier daily.
- If tubing fills with condensate, empty from circuit, not back into the system.

BEST PEEP

Description

Positive end expiratory pressure used with patients on a mechanical ventilator. Allows a preselected pressure to remain in the circuit at end expiration, preventing equilibration of pressure between the atmosphere and the lungs.

Therapeutic Objectives

• To increase pulmonary compliance
• To decrease pulmonary shunt
• To treat refractory hypoxemia

Criteria for Termination

• Improved pulmonary compliance
• Decreased pulmonary shunt
• Improved tissue oxygenation

Contraindications

Compromised hemodynamics

Procedure

1. Evaluate the following parameters:
   a. Blood pressure
   b. Heart rate
   c. Cardiac output
   d. Respiratory rate
2. Institute 3 cm H_2O PEEP and obtain ABG after 20 minutes.
3. Determine tissue delivery of oxygen using the following equation:

$$\text{Tissue delivery} = CO \times CaO_2/100 \text{ ml blood}$$
$$\text{where } CaO_2 = (1.34)(Hb)(sat) + (.003)(PaO_2)$$

4. Vital signs permitting, increase PEEP by 2 to 3 cm H_2O, and repeat the above calculation.
5. If oxygen delivery decreases, best PEEP has been exceeded.
6. Reevaluate vital signs.

Special Considerations

• When levels greater than best PEEP are needed (in some cases to provide an adequate PaO_2 in spite of cardiovascu-

lar compromise), use volume loading and if necessary ionotropic agents and/or vasopressors.
- Closely monitor physiologic parameters to avert possible adverse effects.
- When calculating compliance, subtract PEEP pressures from peak airway and pause pressures.
- Assisted PEEP may be achieved by resetting the zero point for patient inspiratory effort.

Hazards

- Pulmonary barotrauma
- Decreased cardiac output
- Decreased venous return
- Decreased PaO_2 with levels too high
- Increased intracranial pressures
- Decreased compliance

Maintenance

Keep system leak free.

MASK CPAP

Description

Mask CPAP (MCPAP) is positive-pressure therapy applied throughout the respiratory cycle to spontaneously breathing patients via a translucent face mask.

Objectives

- To increase functional residual capacity and PaO_2.
- To decrease work of breathing
- To reduce intrapulmonary shunt
- To avoid tracheal intubation and mechanical ventilation

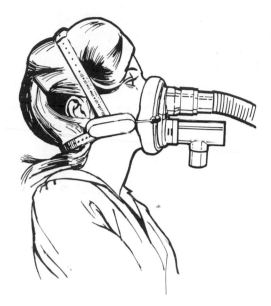

FIG. 6-15. *CPAP mask*

Criteria for Termination

Discontinuation of therapy can be considered when any of the following criteria are met:

- Resolution of the underlying pathological process
- Respiratory rate <30 bpm in previously eucapnic individuals (before MCPAP)
- $PaO_2/FiO_2 > 250$ on minimal CPAP (usually 5 cm H_2O)
- Precipitous rise in $PaCO_2$ necessitating endotracheal intubation and ventilation

Contraindications

- Recent esophageal or gastric anastamosis
- Unstable facial fractures
- Extensive facial lacerations
- Laryngeal trauma

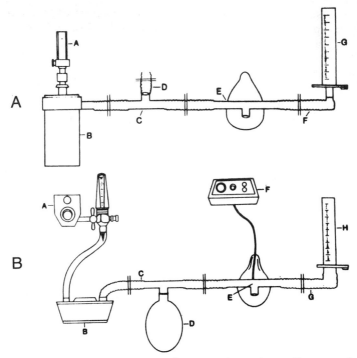

FIG. 6-16. A: *EPAP system (A, flowmeter; B, continuous flow aerosol system; C, T-piece; D, aerosol reservoir; E, patient T-piece with one-way valves; F, expiratory limb; G, threshold resistor).* B: *CPAP system (A, high-flow blender; B, large-volume, low-resistance humidifier; C, inspiratory limb; D, reservoir bag [3–5 liters]; E, patient T-piece; F, high–low pressure alarm and manometer; G, expiratory limb; H, threshold resistor). (Branson RD: Mask CPAP—State of the Art. Resp Care 30(10):849, 1985)*

Procedure

1. Verify physician's order for MCPAP.
2. Evaluate patient's vital signs (BP, HR, RR).
3. Measure minute ventilation if possible.
4. Choose an appropriate CPAP system, CPAP valve, pressure alarm, and mask.
5. Connect air–oxygen sources and adjust FIO_2 according to physician's order.
6. Thoroughly explain the procedure to the patient.
7. Adjust system flow to be, initially, 2 to 3 times the patient's minute ventilation. When V_E cannot be mea-

sured, adjust flow so that, at peak inspiration, system pressure is maintained within 2 cm H_2O of end-expiratory pressure.

8. Attach the mask to the patient using a head strap.
9. Adjust CPAP to appropriate level.
10. Check flow rate to ensure adequate flow to the patient.
11. Auscultate chest and reevaluate vital signs.
12. Adjust low pressure alarm to monitor disconnections.
13. Obtain ABGs after 20 minutes.
14. Increase CPAP in 2 cm to 3 cm H_2O increments until desired PaO_2 is achieved.
15. Continue to monitor ABGs and vital signs.

Hazards

- Aerophagia and gastric distension
- Aspiration of gastric contents
- Decreased cardiac output
- Hypoventilation and CO_2 retention
- Facial skin erosion, erythema
- Patient discomfort

Special Considerations

- Adequately humidify high flows generated in CPAP systems (60–100 liters/minute). Choose a humidifier capable of providing appropriate humidity.
- All CPAP masks should be transparent, lightweight, and possess a soft, pliable, adjustable seal.
- The seal between patient and mask should be effective, but comfortable. Leaks around the mask are permissible as long as system pressure is maintained.
- CPAP valves vary in their performance. A CPAP valve should provide a constant pressure regardless of flow rate.
- The use of a nasogastric tube may be necessary in patients who develop aerophagia and gastric distension.
- Monitor the patient closely for signs of fatigue.
- Continue to monitor vital signs and ABGs.

Maintenance

- Change all tubing and humidifiers daily.
- Inspect masks for leaks and change when necessary.

• Inspect for leaks in order to maintain end-expiratory pressure.

PRESSURE SUPPORT VENTILATION

Pressure support ventilation (PSV) allows the therapist to choose an amount of positive pressure to supplement the patient's spontaneous ventilatory efforts. This augmentation to inspiratory effort usually starts at the initiation of inhalation and ends at a minimum inspiratory flow rate. This new mode of assisted mechanical ventilation has gained enthusiastic support among clinicians managing ventilator patients. Generally, two applications have gained some acceptance. The first uses PSV as assistance to IMV to improve patient tolerance and decrease the work of spontaneous breaths, especially from demand–flow systems. The second uses PSV as a stand–alone ventilatory mode for patients under consideration for weaning. This second application needs further investigation but thoughts are that the PSV mode increases patient comfort as well as

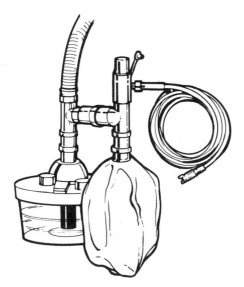

FIG. 6-17. *IMV external setup*

offering an opportunity for endurance muscle training. Most current-generation ventilators have incorporated this new technique.[1]

WEANING

Begin weaning patients from mechanical ventilation only after the patient's physiological parameters suggest that he may be able to support his own ventilation.

The initial problem dictating the patient's need for mechanical ventilation should be reversed or well under control before the weaning process begins.

Malnourishment, a common problem associated with patients requiring mechanical ventilatory support, often plays a role in prolonging the weaning process. Ensure adequate nutrition in those patients expected to be on the ventilator for an extended period of time.

Description

Removal of patients from mechanical ventilation using a systematic approach.

Therapeutic Objectives

To allow physiologic adjustment as well as psychological adjustment in removing the patient from mechanically assisted ventilation.

TABLE 6-6. PHYSIOLOGIC PARAMETERS THAT INDICATE VENTILATORY WEANING

Mechanics	Compliance	> 30 ml/cm H_2O
	Inspiratory force	> -25 cm H_2O
	Vital capacity	> 14 ml/kg body weight
Ventilation	$\dot{V}_D/\dot{V}_T$	< 0.55
	$PaCO_2$	35 mm–45 mm Hg
	pH	$> 7.35, < 7.45$
	Minute ventilation	> 10 l/min
Oxygenation	PaO_2	250 mm–350 mm Hg ($FiO_2 = 1.0$)
	% shunt	$< 15\%$

Criteria for Termination

See Table 6-7.

Contraindications

Unstable cardiovascular or pulmonary system, inadequate ventilatory capability, unstable vital signs.

Procedure

Certain physiologic parameters must be corrected before the patient qualifies for weaning. A general list follows:

1. Acid–base abnormalities
2. Cardiac arrythmias
3. Infection
4. Malnutrition
5. Cardiac output
6. Fluid balance
7. Electrolyte imbalances
8. Shock
9. Level of consciousness
10. Cardiac and pulmonary function. See Table 6-6.

There are two common methods of weaning, IMV and T-tube trials. A third method, HFJV, will be mentioned only for completeness. Dr. Miroslav Klain has had success in weaning ventilator dependent patients using this ventila-

---

TABLE 6-7. CRITERIA FOR REINSTITUTION OF MECHANICAL VENTILATION

Heart Rate	> 110/min or increase of 20/min
ECG	Significant change or arrythmia
Blood pressure	Rise or fall of 20 mm Hg systolic 10 mm Hg diastolic
Respiratory rate	> 35/min or increase of 10/min
PaO_2	> 60 mm Hg
$PaCO_2$	< 55 mm Hg
pH	< 7.35
Pcwp	Increasing

tion mode. To date, however, this mode has not been approved by the FDA and requires a special permit for use.

The first method of weaning, IMV, utilizes the ventilator rate as the weaning tool. The machine rate is gradually lowered to allow more ventilation by the patient, enabling the patient to regulate his own $PaCO_2$. The rate progresses lower until the patient can breath entirely on his own or with a rate of 1 to 2 breaths per minute. The patient can usually be extubated at this time.

PROCEDURE FOR USING IMV

1. Evaluate the physiologic parameters.
2. Change ventilator mode to IMV or SIMV.
3. If an internal IMV system is not available, use an external system.
4. Decrease IMV rate slowly to maintain the desired $PaCO_2$ level
5. Continue to reduce rate observing physiologic parameters.
6. When the IMV rate is between 1 and 3 and the patient stabilizes, you can extubate the patient.

PROCEDURE FOR T-TUBE WEANING

This type of weaning removes the patient from mechanical ventilation for progressively longer periods of time. These trials continue until the patient can maintain an adequate PaO_2 and $PaCO_2$ with spontaneous respirations. Procedure includes the following steps:

1. Evaluate the physiologic parameters.
2. Remove the patient from the ventilator and place on T-tube for 5 to 15 minutes per hour, or as tolerated.
3. Monitor the patient's physiologic status (HR, BP, RR). Should any of these parameters deteriorate the patient should be returned to mechanical ventilation. See Table 6-7.
4. Increase the amount of time the patient is off the ventilator and on the T-tube each hour (watch physiologic parameters).
5. After the patient tolerates a T-tube trial for greater than 1 hour, reevaluate the patient's pulmonary functions (NIF, VC, MVV, RR, HR, BP, ABG).

6. When pulmonary and cardiac function criteria are acceptable, you can extubate the patient.

Special Considerations

- Wean patients only during the waking hours. The patient needs his sleep to maintain his strength.
- Maintain adequate pulmonary hygiene.
- Be sure the patient's nutritional status is sufficient before the weaning process begins.
- Provide psychological support during the weaning process.
- Two IMV systems exist—continuous flow and demand. A demand IMV system provides the spontaneous breaths by opening a valve to provide gas flow between ventilator breaths. The continuous flow IMV system provides a constant flow of gas between ventilator breaths. The patient draws in gas from the continuous flow. Continuous flow takes less effort and the patient consumes less O_2.

Hazards

- Changes in physiologic status
- Failure to wean may cause ventilator dependency

Maintenance

- Give support and encouragement.
- Maintain adequate bronchial hygiene.

MANUAL RESUSCITATOR BAGS

Description

Manual resuscitator bags provide a positive manual-pressure breath to the patient's airway. Originally designed to provide artificial ventilation during lifesaving maneuvers such as CPR, these units are now used whenever a manual positive-pressure breath is needed, as in hyperventilating a patient before and after a suctioning procedure.

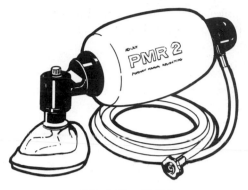

FIG. 6-18. *PMR 2*

Several types on the market today provide the same general result but incorporate different types of valves. These devices may be used with or without a mask to provide ventilation. When used without a mask, the bag is connected directly to either an endotracheal tube or a tracheostomy tube via a standard 15 mm adapter.

The levels of oxygen/air or other gases can be varied depending upon the type of reservoir system. Table 6-8 lists the different types of manual resuscitators, reservoir systems, and valve types currently on the market.

Therapeutic Objectives

- To manually inflate the patient's lungs with positive pressure.
- To provide a means for artificial ventilation in the face of a respiratory emergency.

Criteria for Termination

Mechanical support of ventilation; patient able to adequately maintain spontaneous ventilation.

Contraindications

None; See Hazards.

TABLE 6-8. MANUAL RESUSCITATORS

NAME	PT. VALVE	INLET VALVE	BAG VOL.	MAX F$_I$O$_2$	PRESS. RELIEF
AMBU	Spring disk	Spring disk	2000 ml	Up to 100%	None
Hope	Spring disk	1-way leaf	2000 ml	Up to 100%	Optional magnetic ball 40 cm H$_2$O
Air viva	Spring disk	1-way leaf	2000 ml	Up to 80%	Spring ball set at 40 cm H$_2$O
Hope II	Spring ball	1-way leaf	2000 ml	Up to 100%	Optional magnetic ball 40 cm H$_2$O
AMBU E-2	Diaphragm	1-way leaf	1300 ml	Up to 100%	Stretches at 70 cm H$_2$O
Laerdal RFB-II	Diaphragm & duck bill	1-way leaf	1800 ml	Up to 100%	None
PMR	Diaphragm & leaf	Diaphragm	2000 ml	Up to 80%	None
Air bird	Diaphragm & leaf	1-way leaf	2000 ml	Up to 100%	Fixed orifice leak
Hudson lifesaver	Diaphragm	Leaf	1800 ml	Up to 100%	None
PMR 2	Diaphragm & leaf	Diaphragm	2000 ml	Up to 100%	Optional 40 cm H$_2$O

Procedure

1. Approach the patient and explain procedure when applicable.
2. Obtain the necessary equipment (flowmeter, oxygen tubing, mask, manual resuscitator). *Note:* These pieces of equipment should always be kept together to save time in an emergency!
3. Check integrity of the valve by holding hand over the end of the valve and squeezing the bag. If there is a substantial leak do not use the bag.
4. Adjust flow rate appropriately. Flow rate determines delivered FiO_2 on some units.
5. Attach the unit to the artificial airway if present.
6. If an artificial airway is not in place hold the mask tightly over the patient's nose and mouth. Maintain a patent airway by hyperextending the neck or using the jaw thrust method.
7. Inflate the patient's lungs by squeezing the manual resuscitator with both hands.

Special Considerations

- When using a mask, be sure the airway is patent to prevent insufflation of the stomach.
- Incompetent valves are a hazard to the patient; be sure to check their integrity.
- Use PEEP adapters for those patients supported with mechanical ventilation and PEEP.
- Higher FiO_2s are obtained with a reservoir bag attached to the manual resuscitator.

Hazards

- Hypoxia, hypercarbia with incompetent valves
- Pneumothorax
- Impedance to exhalation when expiratory valve sticks

Maintenance

- Sterilize after each patient use.

REFERENCE

1. MacIntyre NR: Pressure support ventilation. Resp Care 31, No. 3: 189–190, 1986

BIBLIOGRAPHY

Bone RC: Complications of mechanical ventilation and positive end expiratory pressure. Resp Care 27, No. 4: 402–407, 1982

Burton GG, Hodgkin JE (eds): Respiratory Care: A Guide to Clinical Practice. Philadelphia, JB Lippincott, 1984

Carlon G et al: Clinical experience with high frequency jet ventilation. Crit Care Med 9, No. 1: 1–6, 1981

Carlon G, Howland WS, Groeger JS, Ray C, Miodownik S: Role of high frequency jet ventilation in management of respiratory failure. Crit Care Med 12, No. 9: 777–779, 1984

Conception I: ventilatory support in ARDS, Resp Ther, 14, No. 4, 1984

Downs JB: Ventilatory patterns and modes of ventilation in acute respiratory failure. Resp Care 28, No. 5: 586–591, 1983

Ellman H, Dembin H: Lack of adverse hemodynamic effects of PEEP in patients with acute respiratory failure. Crit Care Med 10, No. 11: 706–711, 1982

Gibney RTN, Wilson RS, Pontoppidan H: Comparison of work of breathing with high gas flow and demand valve continuous positive pressure systems. Chest 57:A457, 1982

Hastens RJW, Heenan TJ, Downs JB et al: A comparison of synchronized and nonsynchronized intermittent mandatory ventilation. Resp Care 24:70, 1979

Hudson LD: Cardiovascular complications in acute respiratory failure. Resp Care 28, No. 5: 627–633, 1983

Jaeger MJ, Kurzwes UH, Banner MJ: Transport of gases in high frequency ventilation. Crit Care Med 12, No. 9: 708–710, 1984

Katz JA: PEEP and CPAP in preoperative respiratory care. Resp Ther, Vol. 14, No. 5

Kvetan V, Carlon GC, Howland WS: Acute pulmonary failure in asymmetric lung disease: Approach to management. Crit Care Med 10, No. 2: 114–118, 1982

Lachman B, Jonson B, Lindroth M, Robertson B: Modes of artificial ventilation in severe respiratory distress syndrome. Crit Care Med 10, No. 11: 724–732, 1982

MacIntyre NR: Pressure support ventilation. Resp Care 31, No. 3: 189–190, 1986

Montenegro HD: Complications of mechanical ventilation. Resp Ther 14, No. 5, 1984

Niedermeyer ME, Brigham KL: Prospects for therapeutic interventions in acute respiratory failure. Resp Ther 14, No. 6, 1984

Norlander O: New Concepts of Ventilation. Acta Anaesthesiol Belg 4, Dec 1982

Pace NL, East TD, Westenkow DR, Jordan WS: Differential lung ventilation after unilateral hydrocholoric acid aspiration in the dog. Crit Care Med 11, No. 1: 17–20, 1983

Pierson DJ: Indications for mechanical ventilation in acute respiratory failure. Resp Care 28, No. 5: 570–578, 1983

Shapiro BA, Harrison R, Trout C: Clinical Application of Respiratory Care. Chicago, Year Book Medical Pub, 1979

Sjostrand U: High frequency positive pressure ventilation: A review. Crit Care Med 8, No. 6: 345–364, 1980

Smith JD: Application of mechanical ventilation in acute respiratory failure. Resp Care 28, No. 5: 579–585, 1983

Spearman CB, Sheldon RL (eds): Egans Fundamentals of Respiratory Therapy. St Louis, CV Mosby, 1982

Tahvanainen J, Salmenpera M, Nikki P: Extubation criteria after weaning from intermittent mandatory ventilation and continuous positive airway pressure. Crit Care Med 11, No. 9: 702–707, 1983

monitoring
William DeForge

Monitoring the patient's progress during therapy is perhaps the most important part of respiratory care. The type of monitoring may be as simple as monitoring the patient's pulse during a nebulizer treatment or as complex as observing a rise in the end tidal CO_2 of a mechanically ventilated patient as measured with a sophisticated medical gas mass spectrometer.

The following is a list, albeit partial, of the parameters that should be monitored in determining the efficacy of the therapy modality:

1. FIO_2 delivered
2. Temperature
3. Pulmonary mechanics
4. Bedside pulmonary function
5. Cuff pressures
6. Cardiopulmonary hemodynamics
7. Arterial blood gases
8. Airway pressures
9. Gas volume delivered and exhaled
10. Respirations

This chapter discusses the various types of equipment and procedures used to monitor these parameters. Quick reference charts are also provided.

OXYGEN ANALYZERS

Description

The five different types of oxygen analyzers on the market today are physical, chemical, electrical, electrochemical,

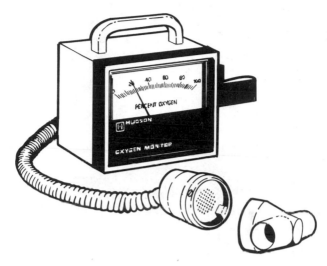

FIG. 7-1. *Paramagnetic oxygen analyzer*

and mass spectrometer. Each uses a different mechanism to analyze the concentration of oxygen.

PHYSICAL ANALYZERS

These devices analyze the FiO_2 using the paramagnetic principle described by Pauling et al. Oxygen (when introduced into a magnetic field) changes the magnetic force design. As the number of oxygen molecules increases in the magnetic field, a mirror attached to a dumbbell rotates and reflects light onto a scale. The greater the number of oxygen molecules present, the greater the degree of rotation of the mirror. The value of FiO_2 is displayed on the scale in either mm Hg or percent. A common example is the Beckman D-2 analyzer.

CHEMICAL ANALYZERS

These devices are usually very accurate for analyzing oxygen. The Scholander unit works by separating carbon dioxide and oxygen and recording the difference in volume. Separation is accomplished by chemically absorbing the CO_2, then the O_2, and measuring the difference. This is the true percentage of oxygen.

ELECTRICAL ANALYZERS

These devices use the principle of thermal conductivity (a Wheatstone bridge) to measure changes of resistance to current flow in a wire. A reference wire is exposed to room air while a second wire is exposed to the gas sample. As the wire is cooled by the gas an increase in current flow occurs. The greater the amount of oxygen, the greater the cooling effect, and thus a higher reading in the FIO_2. The OEM is a common example of this type of analyzer.

ELECTROCHEMICAL ANALYZERS

The first type of electrochemical analyzer, the galvanic fuel cell analyzes FIO_2 by converting oxygen molecules to hydroxyl ions using a hydroxide bath. The bath contains a gold and lead electrode. Hydroxyl ions are formed by absorbing electrons from the gold electrode and then by simple diffusion the ions travel to the lead electrode where they decompose to lead oxide, water, and electrons. This electron current is measured on a meter as a percent of oxygen. Hudson and Biomarine are examples of this type.

The polarographic or Clarke electrode is similar to the galvanic cell except that this type uses batteries to polarize

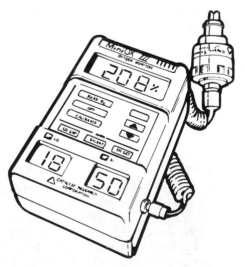

FIG. 7-2. *Galvanic fuel cell oxygen analyzer*

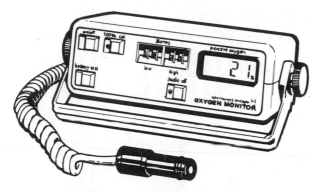

FIG. 7-3. *Polarographic oxygen analyzer*

the electrodes, which gives a better response time. The IL 406 and 407 are examples of this type of analyzer.

MASS SPECTROMETERS

These devices ionize gases and then separate them according to the molecular weight of their ions. A sample of gas drawn into the ionization chamber is bombarded with an electron beam, causing the molecules to lose electrons. A vacuum pump draws the ions into the sampling chamber containing a magnetic field. The ions are deflected downward with the heavier ones falling farther before reaching the collecting plate. The plate counts the number of ions hitting it and determines the relative percentage of the total sample. The Perkin–Elmer, Thoratec and VG are examples of mass spectrometers.

Objectives

To accurately determine the inspired and expired gas mixtures; to clinically evaluate the patient's condition. Accurate FiO_2 measurement is needed for determining pulmonary shunt and interpreting ABGs.

Procedure

1. Turn analyzer off. Using zeroing knob or screw, adjust meter to zero setting.

(*Text continues on p. 240.*)

TABLE 7-1. OXYGEN ANALYZERS

TYPE	TYPICAL BRAND & MODEL	OPERATION	ACCURACY	MAINTENANCE	SPECIAL CONSIDERATIONS
Paramagnetic	Beckman D-2	Insert sample tubing into gas to be measured. Squeeze and release bulb 5–6 times (not necessary in ventilator circuit). Read on flat surface. If reading fluctuates from ventilator cycling, kink hose while reading	±2%	Replace batteries & bulb when they do not function. Replace silica gel when it turns pink	High purchase and repair cost. Safe in flammable atmospheres. Silica crystals should be blue. Halothane will cause false high reading
Chemical	Ametex S-3A/11	CO_2 is absorbed, then O_2 is absorbed. Actual volumetric % is calculated by the difference between the two volumes	±.01%	Replace sensors when out of range	Not affected by partial pressures. Very accurate
Electrical	OEM	Check battery. Place in line with adapter. Read FiO_2	±2%	Replace batteries as needed	

Fuel cell	BioTek model 74223	Is "ON" continuously. Using adapter provided, place in contact with gas to be monitored and read FiO_2	±2%	Replace cell when readings become erratic (100,000 percent-hours is the useful life). Cell should last 9–12 months in normal use.	Easily damaged. Low cost. Can be used in anesthesia. Has high and low alarm limits
Polarographic	Ventronics	Check battery with test button. Insert in line with adapter. Turn on and read with stand on a flat surface	±1%	Replace batteries when battery check indicates they are bad. Replace electrolyte and membrane periodically or when readings are erratic	Not suitable for continuous monitoring since water on membrane may cause erratic readings
Mass spectrometer	Perkin-Elmer VG Gas Analysis Thoratec	The machine removes gas to be analyzed under vacuum	±1%	Professional	Expensive but very versatile. Can measure several gases in different patients sequentially

2. Turn analyzer on. Needle should swing to the 100% setting. Most analyzers indicate a range consistent with a functional battery (i.e., 85% to 100%). Some analyzers use a test control to perform a battery check.
3. If needle does not swing into indicated range, battery should be changed.
4. Expose electrode (probe) to 100% O_2; meter should indicate 100% O_2.
5. If meter does not indicate 100%, adjust with calibration knob.
6. Expose electrode (probe) to room air (21% O_2); meter should indicate 21%.
7. If meter does not indicate 21%, adjust with calibration knob.
8. Repeat steps 4 through 7 until 100% and 21% readings require no adjustment.
9. Frequently, precise calibration of analyzers at 21% and 100% is impossible. If this occurs the following should be observed.

- If the analyzer reads 95% to 100% in 100% O_2 and is accurate at 21% setting, use the analyzer for FiO_2s below 0.50.
- If the analyzer reads 21% to 26% in room air and is accurate at the 100% setting, use the analyzer for FiO_2s above 0.50.
- Remember the accuracy of the analyzer is greater if proper calibration occurs at both the 21% and 100% settings.

Special Considerations

- Perform recalibration every 8 hours at both 21% and 100%.
- Most analyzers directly measure partial pressure of oxygen. At extreme altitude, readjust FiO_2 scale.

Hazards

- Oxygen analyzers that function on the thermal conductivity principle cannot be used in explosive environments and are only accurate in N_2/O_2 mixtures.

• Some analyzers may read inaccurately when used continuously in high absolute humidity or aerosol environments.

Maintenance

• Perform complete calibration at least every 8 hours.
• Perform battery check prior to analyzing a system.
• Change electrode when calibration fails for polarographic analyzer.
• Change fuel cell when calibration fails for galvanic cell analyzer.

TEMPERATURE INDICATORS

Description

Measures the temperature of the gas being inhaled by the patient.

Objective

To deliver the gas as close to body temperature saturated (37°C, 100% relative humidity) as possible in order to eliminate any water loss and drying of secretions in the patient.

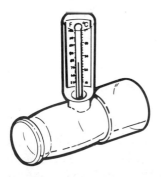

FIG. 7-4. *Temperature indicator*

TABLE 7-2. TEMPERATURE INDICATORS

TYPE	TYPICAL BRAND	ADVANTAGES	DISADVANTAGES
Liquid crystal	Opti-temp	Rugged; accuracy-controlled during manufacture; can be placed very close to patient connection	Color changes are difficult to see in dim light
Thermometer	American Hospital	Low cost; most are easy to read	Liquid can separate if instrument is jarred; in many cases must be placed in manifold, several feet away from patient connection
Thermistor	Bennett Cascade II	Can be used as part of a feedback circuit to control heater output	Needs complicated electronic circuit to be used
Probe	Sensortek	±.01 resolution; A/C, D/C; multiple inputs	Expensive

Procedure

1. Place the device as close to the patient connection as possible since the gas cools about 1°C for each foot of tubing.
2. Check temperature each time ventilator is checked.

Special Considerations

• All devices should be periodically checked for accuracy against a known standard.

Hazards

• None with devices themselves; gas above body temperature can cause respiratory burns, gas below body temperature can cause drying of secretions with the attendant hazards.

Maintenance

• See Table 7-2.

DISCONNECTION ALARMS

Description

An audible and visual indication of equipment malfunction or patient disconnection from equipment.

Objective

To alert the respiratory care practitioner to certain conditions concerning patient care such as disconnection.

Procedure

1. Attach the Bennett volume alarm to the expiratory line; another connection to the ventilator is needed to allow

(*Text continues on p. 246.*)

TABLE 7-3. ALARMS

TYPE	TYPICAL BRAND	USE	ADVANTAGES/ DISADVANTAGES
Volume	Bennett Spirometer Alarm	Adjusted with white stick to within 100 ml of consistently attained tidal volume. Change battery when alarm becomes faint	Measures volume directly
Pressure			
Low only	Bunn LT 40 Bunn LT 50 Healthdyne	Pressure gradient (differential) adjusted so alarm senses about 10 cm H_2O below ventilator cycling pressure	Healthdyne does not usually indicate pressure. Difficult to adjust setting Healthdyne uses batteries; Bunn 120 VAC
High & low	Bunn LT 60 Healthdyne	Bunn is set with selector switches in steps every 10 cm H_2O up to 50 cm H_2O (low) or 60 cm H_2O (high); Healthdyne must be set with continuous range knob	Healthdyne uses batteries; Bunn 120 VAC. Bunn settings frequently several cm H_2O off

I:E ratio	Pneumogard 1230A Mallinckrodt Ventilator Monitor (Bunnell)	Attached to circuit via small-bore tubing. I:E ratio, rate, and inspiratory or expiratory time can be displayed	Pneumogard uses microprocessor for accuracy
Gas O_2 analyzer	Hudson 5590	In-line adapter placed in circuit. High and low limits are set. Membrane is changed every six months or when readings become erratic. Battery checked daily with test button on back	No moisture enters system to affect readings. Accuracy ±1%. Uses polarographic principle
CO_2, O_2, NO_2	SARAcap-Allegheney International	In-line adapter measures CO_2, O_2, NO_2 inspired and end tidal	Continuous display of CO_2 waveform, 24-hour trend. Displays rate and I:E ratio
Ventilation Ventilator monitor	Bunnell-Mallinckrodt Ventilator Alarm	Monitors PEEP, CPAP, rate, PIP, I:E ratios	Has alarm recall. Operates with any conventional ventilator

the spirometer to dump while the ventilator is in the inspiratory phase.
2. Connect pressure alarms to the patient circuit by a piece of small-bore tubing.

Special Considerations

- In patients with extremely high compliance, as in neuro-muscular paralysis or in muscle atrophy, the patient may need only low pressure alarm to monitor disconnection. In this case use volume alarm to monitor adequate ventilation.
- Set time delay to 15 seconds (or more, depending on respiratory rate) so that patient can be suctioned or tubing can be emptied without setting off alarm.

Hazards

- All alarms are only as good as the person who resets them; verify alarm conditions immediately. Do not ignore alarms.
- Excessive false tripping of alarms eventually makes people ignore the alarms.

Maintenance

- Check time delay or volume setting during ventilator check.

SPIROMETERS

Description

Spirometers measure patients' tidal volume, forced vital capacity timed, maximum voluntary ventilation, and slow vital capacity.

Spirometers are of four general types: vortex, vane, rotating cogs, and volume displacement.

With the vortex type, precise struts are placed in a narrow tube to create waves or vortices. An ultrasonic trans-

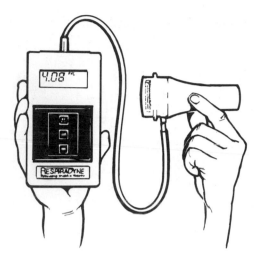

FIG. 7-5. *Pulmonary function spirometer*

ducer produces sound waves that are picked up by a receiver. Each wave or vortex interferes with the sound wave reception and causes a current change. The amount of current change is proportional to a volume. The Bourns LS-75 and the LS-80 are examples of this type.

The Wright Respirometer represents the vane type. With the flow of gas through the device, rotating vanes spin a series of gears indicating volume calibrated in liters on the dial. High (greater than 300 l/min) and low (less than 3 l/min) flow rates cause inaccuracies with this type of spirometer. High flow rates can also damage the vanes.

The Dräger Volumeter is a rotating cog spirometer. Cogs, rather than vanes, rotate to indicate a volume. This meter has a built-in timer for measuring minute volume. Inertia plays a role in the accuracy of this device. High flow rates can also damage this type of spirometer.

The Bennett Monitoring Spirometer is a volume displacement spirometer. As gas enters the unit, a bellows is displaced and the volume is read from a cylinder marked in liters. A calibrated stick in conjunction with an alarm is used to indicate insufficient expired volume.

Peak Flow Meter indicates the Peak Expiratory Flow Rate during an expiratory maneuver.

(*Text continues on p. 250.*)

TABLE 7-4. SPIROMETERS

TYPE	TYPICAL BRAND	ACCURACY	MAINTENANCE	ADVANTAGES/ DISADVANTAGES
Vortex	InterMed	±5%	Remove ultrasonic transducer/detector and dry with alcohol pad if readings become erratic. Keep spare battery pack in charger and change each shift	Display of volume to 1 ml gives false sense of accuracy. Reads flow in either direction. Accurate from 5–250 l/min
Vane	Wright	±5% (assuming 15 l/min minimal flow rate)	Use one-way valve assembly to prevent cross-contamination	Easily damaged if dropped. Accurate only from 20 l–30 l/min flow. May be damaged at flows over 200 l/min
Rotating cog	Dräger	±5%	Use one way valve assembly	Easily damaged
Volume displacement	Bennett Monitoring Spirometer	±50 ml	Remove water when it collects inside	Most accurate. Can accommodate an alarm. Malfunctions easily corrected

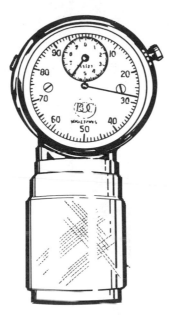

FIG. 7-6. *Wright respirometer*

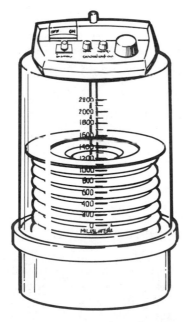

FIG. 7-7. *Monitoring spirometer*

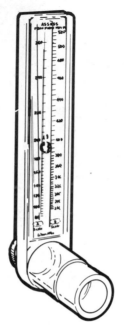

FIG. 7-8. *Peak-flow monitor*

Objectives

To monitor tidal volume to ensure the accurate delivery of volume to the patient; to monitor pulmonary function to assess patient's ventilatory status (FVC, FEV_1); and to monitor change, if any, after a bronchodilator has been administered (SVC).

Procedure

TIDAL VOLUME/MINUTE VENTILATION

1. Attach one-way valves to opposite ends of T-adapter. Setup should ensure unidirectional flow through valves.
2. Attach 5″ flex tube to patient connection port of T-adapter.
3. Attach anatomic mask or Bird 15 mm trach adapter

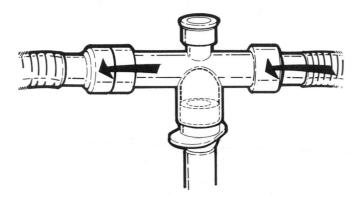

FIG. 7-9. *One-way valve for monitoring*

(dependent on presence of artificial airway) to other end of 5″ flex tube.

4. Attach 15″ flex tube to T-adapter. Gas should flow from T-adapter through 15″ flex tube.

5. Attach other end of 15″ flex tube to spirometer.

6. Determine and record vital signs, pulse, BP, temperature, and respiratory rate.

7. Instruct patient to breathe normally. Apply mask to face or attach to artificial airway. For a cooperative patient, a mouthpiece may be used in place of the anatomic mask. When using a mouthpiece, apply a nose clip to prevent leaks.

8. Measure volume exhaled for ten breaths and determine average tidal volume.

9. Multiply tidal volume by respiratory rate to determine minute volume or measure for one full minute.

VITAL CAPACITY

1. Complete steps 1 to 6 (Tidal Volume/Minute Ventilation).

2. Attach spirometer by way of the mask, Bird 15 mm adapter, or mouthpiece and nose clip. After deep inspiration have patient exhale as much as possible (slowly for SVC, forcefully for FVC). Repeat three times, recording largest volume.

TABLE 7-5. BEDSIDE PULMONARY FUNCTIONS

TYPE	PROCEDURE	RESULTS
Forced vital capacity	Patient should have procedure explained before being placed on device. Nose clips should be placed on his nose and he should be instructed to seal his lips tightly around the mouthpiece. After about 1 minute of tidal ventilation to accustom him to the equipment, instruct him to take as deep a breath as possible, hold it for a short period, and then exhale as hard as possible for as long as he can. Repeat 3 times and use best effort in calculations	Use predicted normal from a nomogram (such as Cory). If value is ±20% of predicted, it is considered WNL. Decreased values appear in restrictive disease with normal $FEV_1/FVC\%$ and in obstructive disease with decreased $FEV_1/FVC\%$ Units: ml FVC should be >12 ml/kg for weaning
$\dfrac{FEV_1}{FVC\%}$	Take the volume of air in first second of forced vital capacity (FEV_1). Divide this by the FVC measured above and express as a percentage	Using actual FEV_1 and FVC, normal for 20-year-old male is 83% and decreases approximately 2% for every 10 years. Although there are tables for normal FEV_1, they are essentially worthless since they are not related to FVC. For example, if the FVC is decreased, the FEV_1 will certainly be decreased but, as a percent of FVC, may be normal. The value is a gross indicator of airways obstruction

Special Considerations

• Each patient should have his own one-way valve assembly to prevent cross-contamination when monitoring more than one patient.

Hazards

• Patients on FiO_2 greater than .21 or on PEEP may become hypoxic when removed from the oxygen source. Monitor closely.

CUFF PRESSURE MEASUREMENT

Description

Determination of pressure exerted by tracheal tube cuff on wall of trachea.

Objective

To maintain pressure on the wall of the trachea under 20 mm to 25 mm Hg, allowing capillary blood flow and preventing tissue necrosis.

Procedure

"ALL THE REST"

1. Plug the stopcock into the pilot tube.
2. Once you establish minimal occluding volume (MOV, no-leak) or minimal leak (ML), turn the stopcock to connect manometer to cuff. Read pressure.

BIVONA

1. Once tube has been inserted, withdraw all air with a syringe.
2. Clamp the pilot port and release the syringe.
3. Using the volume in ml, the pressure on the trachea is read from the graph. See Airway Management in Chapter 5.

The cuff pressure in the rest of the tubes, regardless of design differences, is measured in the same manner. (Bivona uses a unique method to estimate pressure.)

Special Considerations

• If the pilot tube on a Bivona tube is accidentally removed, the cuff can still be deflated by cutting off the tip of a 19- or 20-gauge needle and inserting the needle into the hole to deflate the cuff.
• See Chapter 5 for additional considerations.

Hazards

• Cuff may become partially deflated, allowing secretions to enter trachea.
• High cuff pressure can result in necrosis, fibrosis and, ultimately, tracheal stenosis, a severe complication.

NEGATIVE INSPIRATORY FORCE

Description

Negative inspiratory force has been used to evaluate pulmonary mechanics. By having the patient inhale against an occlusion negative inspiratory force is generated.

Objective

To evaluate patient's ability to generate negative inspiratory pressure. Normal adult values are 75 cm to 100 cm H_2O.

Procedure

1. Attach manometer to anatomic mask or Bird adapter.
2. Attach setup to patient, allowing patient to breathe normally by way of the vent in the manometer system.
3. At the end of a normal exhalation, occlude vent in manometer system.
4. Observe NIF manometer and continue procedure for no more than 20 seconds.

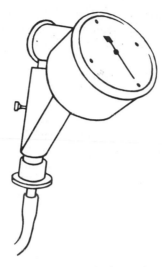

FIG. 7-10. *Pressure manometer attached to endotracheal tube for determination of negative inspiratory force.*

5. Record greatest negative pressure generated and length of time vent is occluded.

Special Considerations

• Reinstitute mechanical ventilation immediately following procedure.
• Reinstitute supplemental oxygenation immediately following procedure.

TABLE 7-6. MEASUREMENT OF INSPIRATORY FORCE

NAME	METHOD	COMMENTS
Inspiratory force	Use manometer (such as Boehringer inspiratory force gauge) with adapter on tracheal tube or mask on face. Use device with open port that can be manually occluded when force is measured and left open between measurements	Units: cm H_2O. Normal: >-70. For weaning, should be >-25

Hazards

- Hypoxemia
- Cardiovascular instability
- Cross-contamination

Maintenance

- Flex tubing, Briggs adapter, mask, and mouthpiece should be for single-patient use.
- Spirometer and NIF manometer should be cleaned with alcohol between patients.
- Accuracy of equipment should be evaluated weekly.

HEART RATE/RESPIRATORY RATE MONITORS

Description

The use of heart rate and respiratory rate monitors is crucial in the management of the critically ill patient. Heart rate monitors sense the electrical depolarization and repolarization of the heart and display the heart rate on a meter or digital display. Most respiratory rate monitors (impedance pneumographs) are attached by way of chest electrodes that sense the changes in impedance as the thoracic cage expands and contracts during ventilation.

Objectives

To monitor heart and respiratory rate; to alert medical personnel to changes in patient's cardiac and respiratory rate.

Procedure

HEART RATE

1. Place electrodes or limb leads on patient according to monitor specifications.
2. Attach leads to monitor and turn on.

3. Auscultate heartbeat and adjust sensitivity until the heart rate indicator light or a QRS pattern appears with each heart beat.
4. If monitor has QRS display, adjust gain control until QRS is easily distinguishable in size.
5. Set high and low heart rate alarm settings.

RESPIRATORY RATE

1. Place electrodes on patient according to monitor directions. Make sure noticeable movement exists as electrodes move away from each other with every breath.
2. Connect leads to monitor and turn on.
3. Adjust sensitivity until breath indicator is activated with each breath.
4. Set delay for apnea alarm (15 or 30 seconds).
5. Set high and low respiratory rate alarm.

Special Considerations

• Electrodes must be wet to sense heart rate and respiratory rate appropriately.
• An impedance pneumograph respiratory rate monitor will not sense obstructive apnea if the patient makes respiratory movements.
• Obese patients, and those with barrel chests, sometimes have high impedance and the unit will fail to sense all respiratory efforts.
• Alarms must be set properly to ensure adequate monitoring capabilities.
• Diaphoretic patients may need to have the electrodes changed often.
• Failure of electrode to remain on the chest will cause an alarm condition; do not merely silence the alarm, verify the alarm condition.

MEAN AIRWAY PRESSURE MONITORING

Mean airway pressure (MAP) is determined by calculating the area under the curve produced during the respiratory cycle. Changes in the peak airway pressure, I : E ratio, or PEEP affect MAP.

The mean pressure of the entire cycle is the arithmetic average of an infinite number of points under the curve. The greater the number of points averaged, the more accurate the reading will be. See Fig. 7-11. Calculation of the mean area of an irregular curve is obtained by using mathematic calculus or electronic calculators.

Recent data have suggested that mean airway pressure may reflect respiratory and cardiovascular functions. Electronic monitors are available for the accurate monitoring of mean airway pressure.

Equipment

1. Pressure monitor
2. T–adapter
3. Small–bore tubing

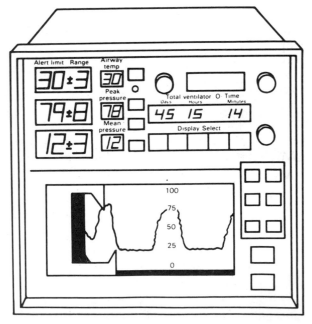

FIG. 7-11. *Respiratory parameter monitor, capable of monitoring mean airway pressure, FiO₂, peak airway pressure, and other parameters.*

Procedure

1. Calibrate the monitor to the manufacturer's specifications.
2. Attach the adapter to the ventilator circuit as close to the patient's airway as possible.
3. Attach the small-bore tubing from the pressure outlet of the monitor to the adapter in the ventilator circuit.
4. Set the monitor to read out the calculated mean airway pressure.

Maintenance

• Check the monitor calibration every 4 to 8 hours.
• Change the adapter system each time the ventilator circuit is changed.

Hazards

• Failure to calibrate the monitor correctly may lead to inappropriate ventilator changes because of inaccurate mean airway pressure readouts.
• Disconnection from the small-bore tubing causes a leak in the ventilator circuit which may impair patient oxygenation (especially with patients on PEEP).

PULMONARY MECHANIC/VENTILATION FORMULAS

Description

Measurement and calculation of pulmonary parameters directly related to lung function and disease.

Objectives

To assess patient's clinical condition, whether he is improving or deteriorating, and whether ministrations are actually helping him.

(*Text continues on p. 264.*)

TABLE 7-7A. PULMONARY MEASUREMENT PROCEDURES

NAME	METHOD	COMMENTS
Compliance	Using inspiratory hold (or temporarily occluding the exhalation valve), determine equilibration pressure. Multiply equilibration pressure by circuit compliance factor. Subtract from tidal volume set. Then divided by plateau pressure	Decreases in most disease entities. Used to determine best PEEP
Resistance	Subtract plateau pressure from peak cycling pressure. Divide by average inspiratory flow rate	Increases in some chronic diseases (asthma, bronchitis)
$\dot{V}_D : \dot{V}_T$ ratio	For the estimate (which is quite close to the measured), use a Radford nomogram for $\dot{V}_E$ (est.) and measure $\dot{V}_E$. For the measured value, mean $PECO_2$ must be measured with a capnograph and arterial ABG obtained.	Units: None. Normal: 0.33. For weaning should be <0.55

TABLE 7-7B. PULMONARY MECHANIC AND VENTILATION FORMULAS

	ABBREVIATION	FORMULA	RANGE	NORMAL
V_T	Tidal volume		0.4–1.5 liter	0.5–1 liter
f	Respirations per minute		6–30 bpm	6–18 bpm
Comp volume	Compressible volume		1–5 ml/cm	3 ml/cm
Plat pressure	Plateau pressure		20–80 cm H_2O*	
PIP	Peak inspiratory pressure		10–100 cm H_2O	
PEEP	Positive end expiratory pressure		0–50 cm H_2O	
P_ECO_2	Partial pressure of expired carbon dioxide		10–100 mm Hg	30–50 mm Hg
$PaCO_2$	Partial pressure of arterial carbon dioxide		10–75 mm Hg*	35–45 mm Hg
del V_T	Delivered tidal volume	del $V_T = V_T - (PIP \times Comp\ vol)$ PIP = peak inspiratory pressure Comp vol = compressible volume	0.2–1.4 liter*	6–8 ml/kg ideal body weight
$\dot{V}_E$	Minute ventilation	$\dot{V}_E = V_T \times f$ $\dot{V}_E$ = minute volume (l/min) V_T = tidal volume f = respirations per minute	2–50 lpm*	2–7 lpm (60 ml/kg/min)

(Continued)

TABLE 7-7B. PULMONARY MECHANIC AND VENTILATION FORMULAS (Continued)

	ABBREVIATION	FORMULA	RANGE	NORMAL
D comp	Dynamic compliance	$Cdyn\ eff = \dfrac{V_T}{(PIP - PEEP)}$ $Cdyn\ eff_T$ = effective total respiratory dynamic compliance (l/ cm H_2O) V_T = tidal volume PIP = peak inspiratory pressure $PEEP$ = positive end expiratory pressure	0–1 liter/cm H_2O	0.1 liter/cm H_2O
St comp	Static compliance	$C\ eff_T = \dfrac{V_T}{(P_{PLT} - PEEP)}$ $C\ eff_T$ = effective total respiratory static compliance (l/ cm H_2O) V_T = tidal volume P_{PLT} = proximal airway plateau pressure $PEEP$ = positive end expiratory proximal airway pressure	0–1 liter/cm H_2O	0.2 liter/cm H_2O
$\dot{V}_D$	Dead space volume	$\dot{V}_D = \dfrac{\dot{V}_E(PaCO_2 - P_ECO_2)}{PaCO_2 - PiCO_2}$ $\dot{V}_D$ = ventilation per minute of the physiological dead space $\dot{V}_E$ = minute ventilation $PaCO_2$ = partial pressure of arterial carbon dioxide	0–150 ml	2 ml/kg ideal body weight

Symbol	Description	Definition		
		P_E = partial pressure of expired carbon dioxide P_I = partial pressure of inspired carbon dioxide		
$\dot{V}_D/\dot{V}_T$	Dead space to tidal volume ratio	$V_D/V_T = \dfrac{PaCO_2 - PeCO_2}{PaCO_2}$ $PaCO_2$ = partial pressure of arterial carbon dioxide $PeCO_2$ = partial pressure of mixed expired carbon dioxide	0.15–3.5 ml*	.25–.3 ml/kg ideal body weight
$\dot{V}_A$	Alveolar ventilation	$\dot{V}_A = f(V_T - V_D)$ $\dot{V}_A$ = alveolar ventilation (lpm) f = breathing frequency V_T = tidal volume V_D = dead space	1–7 lpm*	1–5 lpm
IF	Inspiratory force		0–120 mm Hg*	>−70 (normal) >−25 (weaning)
R_T	Resistance	$R_T = (PIP - P_{PLT})/\dot{V}_I$ R_T = total respiratory resistance (cm H_2O/l/sec) PIP = peak inspiratory pressure P_{PLT} = plateau pressure $\dot{V}_I$ = inspiratory flow rate $Raw = \Delta P_{AW} - P_A/\Delta\dot{V}$ Raw = airway resistance (cm H_2O/l/sec) Paw = proximal airway pressure P_A = alveolar pressure		1.1–1.9 cm H_2O/liter/sec

* On constant flow generator

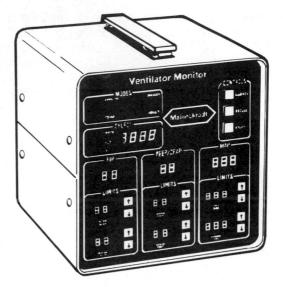

FIG. 7-12. *Ventilator monitor*

Procedure

See Table 7-7A.

Special Consideration

See Table 7-7A.

Hazards

See Table 7-7A.

HEMODYNAMIC MONITORING

Description

The development of the flow-directed pulmonary artery catheter by Swan and Ganz has made therapeutic intervention in cases of critically ill patients more definitive.

The Swan–Ganz catheter is inserted through a large vein and advanced through the right atrium, right ventricle, and finally into the pulmonary artery. With the balloon inflated, the catheter will drift with the flow of blood until it causes an occlusion. At this point the catheter is in the pulmonary capillary wedge position. Pressures here reflect the pressures in the left side of the heart (left heart filling pressures), indicating left ventricular function.

The catheter has three separate ports. The distal port, at the very end of the catheter, rests in the pulmonary artery and usually has a thermistor on the end for thermodilution cardiac output determinations. A second, proximal port rests in the superior vena cava. Usually this port is used for infusion of fluids and cold fluids for cardiac output determinations. This port can also be used to measure the central venous pressure. A third port is used for the inflation of the balloon, located at the distal end of the catheter. Figure 7-13 shows the common waveforms and normal pressure ranges.

The Swan–Ganz catheter allows for monitoring of central venous pressures, cardiac output, fluid balance, pulmonary artery pressure, and left ventricular function. It also allows one to obtain true mixed venous blood for determination of intrapulmonary shunt.

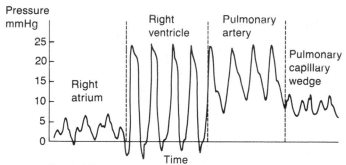

Normal Pressures

Right atrium — 0-6 mmHg
Right ventricle — 20-30/0-5 mmHg
Pulmonary artery — 20-30/< 12 mmHg
Pulmonary capillary wedge — 6-15/4-12 mmHg

FIG. 7-13. *Swan–Ganz pressure display*

TABLE 7-8A. HEMODYNAMIC MONITORING

FUNCTION	PROCEDURE	NORMAL	COMMENTS
Pulmonary artery pressure	Continuously monitored on oscilloscope (CRT screen) for hemodynamics; diastolic (PAD) can be close to LA pressure (but is not always). Mean pressure used for calculating pulmonary vascular resistance	25/10-12; mean: Normal 15–18 mm Hg; PVR: 150–250 dyne cm/sec^{-5}	PVR is calculated as *pressure flow* If units of mm Hg/l/min are used, normal is 1.5–2.0. If mm Hg/ml/ sec are used, normal is 0.1
Pulmonary capillary wedge pressure	Balloon at tip of catheter is inflated (volume is stated on port for syringe) for less than one minute. Waveform should change to PCWP. Mean pressure is read	5–15 mm Hg mean	Abbreviations include Paw, Pcw, Pao.
Central venous pressure	Monitored on oscilloscope or water manometer. Height of manometer or transducer for oscilloscope is vital; should be at level of right atrium	0–6.7 mm Hg	It is useful to mark a line on the side of the chest so that each reading is made at the same level
Cardiac output	Following instructions with cardiac output computer (made by KMA, Edwards Labs, and Instrumentation Labs), push start button and rapidly inject 10 ml	Minimum 2.5 l/min/M^2; cardiac index $= \dfrac{CO}{BSA}$	Can be repeated every minute if necessary. Runs 7% higher than Fick but provides reproducible results

Intrapulmonary shunt	$\dfrac{CcO_2 - CaO_2}{CcO_2 - C\bar{v}O_2}$	Determine arterial content from arterial blood gas. Determine mixed venous content from pulmonary artery sample. For capillary content, assume P_AO_2 saturation = 1.0 and calculate hemoglobin saturation and dissolved oxygen	Units: Percent, Normal: <5. Used to determine optimal PEEP.
A–$\bar{v}O_2$ difference	$CaO_2 - C\bar{v}O_2$	See shunt above	Units: ml O_2/dl blood. Normal: 4–5. If increases, cardiac output is insufficient for tissue demands
Systemic vascular resistance*	$SVR = \dfrac{(MAP - CVP)\ (79.9)}{CO}$	Determine left ventricular afterload. MAP = mean systemic blood pressure, $\dfrac{(systole\text{-}diasystole)}{3}$ + diastole; CVP = central venous pressure CO = cardiac output	Units: dyne/sec/cm^{-5}. Normal: 900–1200
Pulmonary vascular resistance*	$PVR = \dfrac{(\bar{PAP} - Pcwp)(79.9)}{CO}$	Determine right ventricular afterload. $\bar{PAP}$ = mean pulmonary artery pressure; Pcwp = Pulmonary capillary wedge pressure; CO = cardiac output	Units: dyne/sec/cm^{-5}. Normal: 400

* Osgood CF, Watson MH, Slaughter MS, and MacIntyre NR: Hemodynamic monitoring in respiratory care. Resp Care 29: 1, 1984

TABLE 7-8B HEMODYNAMIC PARAMETERS AND FORMULAS

ABBREVIATION		FORMULA	RANGE	NORMAL
CO	Cardiac output	$Q(CO) = \dfrac{\dot{V}O_2}{CaO_2 - CvO_2 \times 10}$ $\dot{V}O_2$ = ml/min STPD CaO_2 = arterial O_2 content (ml/100 ml) CvO_2 = mixed venous O_2 content (ml/100 ml) $\dot{Q}$ = heart rate (HR) × stroke volume (SV)	1–8.5 liter	4–8 liter (adults)
MAP	Mean arterial pressure	$MAP = \dfrac{(systolic - diastolic) + diastolic}{3}$	40–180 mm Hg	82–102 mm Hg (adults)
PCWP	Pulmonary capillary wedge pressure		5–15 mm Hg	
PAP	Pulmonary artery pressure		6–25 mm Hg	6–18 mm Hg
CVP	Central venous pressure		2–25 mm Hg	0.7–6.7 mm Hg
SBP	Systolic blood pressure		40–200 mm Hg	100–140 mm Hg

BSA	Body surface area	$BSA(m^2) = wt^{0.425} \times Ht^{0.725} \times 0.00781$	1–3.5 m²	
SV	Stroke volume	$SV = \dfrac{CO \times 100}{HR}$ CO = cardiac output (l/min) HR = heart rate	60–90 ml/beat*	60–130 ml/beat
SI	Stroke index		40–60 ml/beat/m²	30–50 ml/beat/m²
CI	Cardiac index	$CI = CO/BSA$ CO = cardiac output (l/min) BSA = body surface area (m²)	3–3.4 liter/min/m²*	2.7–4.5 liter/min/m²* (children and adults)
LVSWI	Left ventricular stroke work index	$LVSWI = SI \times (MAP - PAWP) \times 0.0136$ SI = stroke index (ml/m²) MAP = mean arterial pressure (mm Hg) PAWP = pulmonary artery wedge pressure (mm Hg)	45–60 g · m/m²	42–64 g · m/m²
RVSWI	Right ventricular stroke work index	$RVSWI = SI \times MPAP - CVP) \times 0.0136$ SI = stroke index MAP = mean arterial pressure (mm Hg) CVP = central venous pressure (mm Hg)	5–10 g · m/m²*	3.8–7.6 g · m/m² (children and adults)
SVRI	Systemic vascular resistance index	$SVRI = \dfrac{MAP - CVP}{CI}$ MAP = mean arterial pressure (mm Hg) CVP = central venous or mean right arterial pressure (mm Hg) CI = cardiac index (l/min/m²)	1970–2398 dyne · sec/cm⁵/m²*	1760–2600 dyne · sec/cm⁵/m²

(Continued)

269

TABLE 7-8B HEMODYNAMIC PARAMETERS AND FORMULAS (Continued)

	ABBREVIATION	FORMULA	RANGE	NORMAL
PVRI	Pulmonary vascular resistance index	$PVRI = \dfrac{MPAP - PAWP}{CI}$ MPAP = mean pulmonary artery pressure (mm Hg) PAWP = pulmonary artery wedge pressure or mean left arterial pressure (mm Hg) CI = cardiac index (l/min/m²)	255–285 dyne · sec/cm⁵/m⁵*	45–255 dyne · sec/cm⁵/m⁵
TI	Triple index	$TI = SBP \times HR \times PCWP$ SBP = systolic blood pressure HR = heart rate PCWP = pulmonary capillary wedge pressure	60,000–180,000	120,000
RPP	Rate pressure product	$RPP = HR \times SBP$ HR = heart rate SBP = systolic blood pressure	12,000	9600–14,000
CaO_2	Oxygen content	$CaO_2 = (Hb \times 1.39 \times O_2sat) + (0.0031 \times PaO_2)$		
CvO_2	Mixed venous oxygen content	$CvO_2 = (Hb \times 1.39 \times O_2sat) + (0.0031 \times PvO_2)$ $CcO_2 = (Hb \times 1.39 \times O_2sat) + (0.0031 \times PcO_2)$		
$\dot{Q}_s/\dot{Q}_T$	Venous to arterial shunt	$\dot{Q}_s/\dot{Q}_T = \dfrac{CcO_2 - CaO_2}{CcO_2 - CvO_2}$	1%–100%	2%–5%

$\dot{Q}_s$ = shunted portion of cardiac output
Q_T = total cardiac output
CcO_2 = oxygen content of end pulmonary blood (ml/100 ml)
CaO_2 = oxygen content of arterial blood (ml/100 ml)
$C\bar{v}O_2$ = mixed venous oxygen content (ml/100 ml)

$C(a-\bar{v})O_2$	Arteriovenous oxygen difference	$C(a-\bar{v})O_2 = CaO_2 - C\bar{v}O_2$ CaO_2 = arterial oxygen content $C\bar{v}O_2$ = mixed venous oxygen content	4–6 vol%*	4.5–6 vol%
O_2AV	Oxygen availability	$O_2AV = CaO_2 \times CI \times 10$ CaO_2 = arterial oxygen content (ml/100 ml) CI = cardiac index (l/min/m²)	500–800 ml/min/m²*	520–720 ml/min/m²
$\dot{V}O_2$	Oxygen consumption	$\dot{V}O_2 = (CaO_2 - C\bar{v}O_2) \times CI \times 10$ CaO_2 = arterial oxygen content $C\bar{v}O_2$ = mixed venous oxygen content CI = cardiac index	100–300 ml/min/m²*	120–250 ml/min/m²
$\dot{V}O_2/I$	Oxygen consumption index	$\dot{V}O_2/I = \dot{V}O_2/BSA$ $\dot{V}O_2$ = oxygen consumption BSA = body surface area	100–180 ml/min/m²	
O_2ER	Oxygen extraction ratio	$O_2ER = \dfrac{(CaO_2 - C\bar{v}O_2) \times 100}{CaO_2}$ CaO_2 = arterial oxygen content $C\bar{v}O_2$ = mixed venous oxygen content	.01%–1%	.22%–.3%

* On constant flow generator

Objectives

To accurately assess the patient's cardiopulmonary status and fluid balance.

Procedure

Note: The catheter should be inserted by a physician, using aseptic technique, into a large vein. The following steps are involved:

1. Attach distal lumen of catheter to heperanized saline solution with pressure bag and transducer. Flush through sampling stopcock.
2. Attach proximal lumen of catheter to flush solution.
3. Insert catheter using aseptic technique.
4. Attach 1 ml syringe to balloon port.
5. At the level of the right atrium, inflate the balloon and advance across the tricuspid valve to the right ventricle, then across the pulmonic valve into the pulmonary artery.
6. Advance the catheter until you see a change in the pressure waveform.
7. Deflate the balloon. The waveform should change back to that of the pulmonary artery (Fig. 7-11).

Special Considerations

- *Important:* Use aseptic technique.
- Monitor closely for arrhythmias during insertion.
- Change dressing and clean insertion site daily.
- Monitor patients on high levels of PEEP with a pulmonary artery catheter in place.
- Changes in pleural pressure affect the pressure waveform.

Hazards

- Overinflation of the balloon can cause rupture of the pulmonary artery.
- Embolism
- Sepsis

- Iatrogenic pulmonary infarction
- Arrhythmias

Maintenance

- Distal port should be maintained with a pressure bag, intraflo device, and dome assembly. A solution of 1000 USP units of sodium heparin and 500 ml normal saline should be infused through this line.
- Proximal port should be maintained with an infusion pump and solution of the physician's choice.
- Change solution in pressure bag, intraflo device, and dome at least every 48 hours.

OXIMETRIX BALLOON-TIPPED FLOW-DIRECTED PULMONARY ARTERY CATHETER

Description

The Oximetrix uses three wavelengths of light in the red and infrared spectrum to measure the saturation of blood. This is done by measuring the amount of relative absorption of light by hemoglobin and oxyhemoglobin by spectrophotometry.

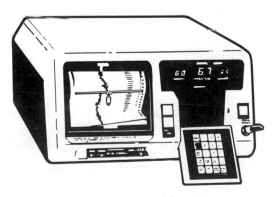

FIG. 7-14. *Catheter oximetry*

Objective

To obtain continuous readings of saturation from arterial or mixed venous sources for monitoring the progress of the patient.

Procedure

1. Determine the need for pulmonary artery catheterization.
2. Obtain informed consent.
3. Press the RUN switch, WARM UP message will be displayed.
4. Lower the keyboard and enter the desired HI and LOW saturation limits.
5. Press ART/VEN key to display ARTERIAL or VENOUS for arterial or pulmonary artery catheter respectively.
6. Peel back the outer wrapping, leaving the catheter still covered by the inner wrap.
7. Place the optical module in the catheter tray.
8. Place the optical connector from the catheter into the optical module receptacle.
9. Turn on the recorder by pressing the RECORD INT and the 4 INCHES PER HOUR keys.
10. Press PUSH on the catheter optical reference assembly.
11. Press STANDARDIZE; the display should read STANDARDIZE AND CATH PREPARED? PRESS ENTER.
12. If the optical reference has been pushed, press the ENTER key.
13. After 20 seconds "500" or "501" should appear in the display window.
14. If it does not, repeat the steps above; if it does, then the catheter is ready for insertion.
15. Use hospital procedure for insertion of pulmonary artery catheters.
16. Press the 1 INCH PER MINUTE key during insertion.

17. After the catheter is in the proper position, press the INT REPRG key.

IN VIVO CALIBRATION

Indicated when the catheter has not been standardized before insertion or when a calibration against a laboratory value is desired.

1. Press the DRAW BLOOD key.
2. Clear the distal line and draw the blood sample.
3. Measure oxygen hemoglobin saturation in the blood gas lab.
4. Enter the analyzed saturation value and press ENTER.
5. Press OPERATE if the value is correct. If value is incorrect, press CLEAR SAT and reenter the value.

Special Considerations

- Kinks in the catheter will cause inaccurate readings; the message LOW LIGHT CHECK CATH will appear, indicating possible damage to the catheter.
- Proper warm-up time is essential for accuracy. If main module is left unplugged for more than 4 hours, 72 hours may be required for warm-up; if unplugged for less than 4 hours, 15 minutes should be sufficient.
- The message EEE indicates an abnormal condition and the service representative should be notified.
- The message --- indicates saturation out of range, possibly from equipment loss of memory, improper standardization, or optical module malfunction.

Hazards

- Hazards associated with the insertion of a pulmonary artery catheter (pneumothorax, sepsis, etc.).

Maintenance

- Keep the optical connector free from dirt and debris.
- Keep the air filter clean.

CAPNOGRAPHY

Description

Capnography allows the clinician to continuously monitor exhaled CO_2. The peak exhaled CO_2 correlates well with arterial CO_2 in patients with normal ventilation/perfusion ratios.

Most capnographs measure CO_2 concentration by measuring the absorption of an infrared beam by the gas mixture. As the CO_2 concentration changes, so does the level of absorption.

The capnograph can be used on either mechanically ventilated or spontaneously ventilating patients. The monitor employs a vacuum device that withdraws a gas sample from the patient's inspired/expired gas. Carbon dioxide concentration is displayed digitally or on an x–y chart recorder.

Objectives

To continuously monitor exhaled carbon dioxide and to assess the adequacy of ventilation.

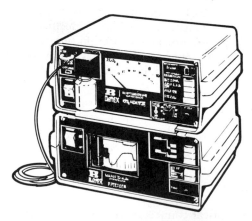

FIG. 7-15a. *End tidal CO_2 monitor*

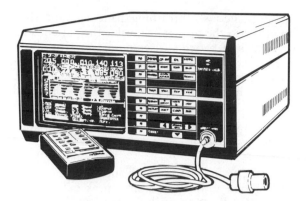

FIG. 7-15b.   *Monitoring expired gases (SARA)*

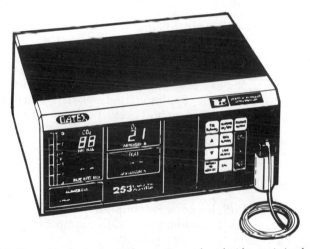

FIG. 7-15c.   *Monitoring expired gases. (Reproduced with permission from Shapiro BA, Harrison RA, Walton JR: Clinical Application of Blood Gases, 3rd ed. Copyright © 1982 by Year Book Medical Publishers, Inc., Chicago)*

Procedure

1. Perform a two-point calibration of the monitor using a known high and low CO_2 gas concentration.
2. Attach sampling line to patient.

- For spontaneously breathing patients, tape the sampling tube so the tip sits just inside the patient's nostril.
- For intubated patients, use an adapter that allows the patient's exhaled gas to be sampled. In IMV systems, a sterile sampling tube may need to be advanced into the ET or trach tube for proper monitoring of true exhaled gas.

3. Adjust sampling flow rate. Start at 30 ml/min and slowly increase until you see a "plateau" on the exhaled CO_2 curve.
4. If available, set the desired high and low alarm settings 5 mmHg above and below desired peak exhaled PCO_2.
5. Draw a blood gas to evaluate the correlation of peak exhaled and arterial PCO_2.

Special Considerations

- An increase in a–$ADCO_2$ is to be expected in situations in which there is ventilation in excess of perfusion (*i.e.,* hypovolemia, shock, pulmonary hypertension, pulmonary embolus, and bronchopulmonary dysplasia). When there is an a–$ADCO_2$ gradient and peaked exhaled CO_2 is less than arterial CO_2, the monitor may still be used to monitor the trending of arterial CO_2.

Hazards

- Obstruction of airway with sampling tube
- Inaccurate V_ECO_2 reading if monitor, sampling flow, or tubing is adjusted inappropriately
- Overinflation of balloon may cause pulmonary artery rupture

Maintenance

- Recalibrate the capnograph to two known CO_2 gas concentrations every 8 hours.
- Clear the sampling tubing of moisture and mucus as necessary. Some monitors have H_2O traps built into the system.

• Change the sampling tubing every 24 hours and between patients.

EAR OXIMETRY

Description

Ear oximetry measures the arterial oxygen saturation of blood noninvasively. Saturation is obtained by measuring the amount of light that is reflected from two wavelengths in the vascular bed of the ear lobe.

Objective

To obtain arterial oxygen saturation by a noninvasive technique, to monitor the oxygenation status of the patient during the weaning process, and to monitor the oxygenation status of the patient during sleep apnea, exercise, pulmonary function studies, etc.

Procedure

1. Approach the patient and explain the procedure.
2. Plug in the ear oximeter and allow for adequate warm-up time
3. Calibrate if necessary according to the manufacturer's specifications.
4. Vasodilate the earlobe by rubbing vigorously with an alcohol swab.

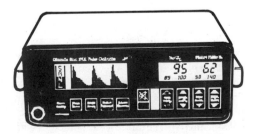

FIG. 7-16. *Pulse oximeter*

5. Attach the ear probe to the earlobe and allow a few minutes for equilibration before reading the saturation.

Special Considerations

• May be inaccurate in patients with dark pigmentation, elevated bilirubins, or COHgb levels above 4%.
• An arterial sample should be obtained to ensure correlation between the actual arterial saturation and the ear oximeter reading.
• Adequate warm-up time is needed before readings are recorded.
• Inaccuracies may result at saturation readings below 80%.
• At the high end of the oxyhemoglobin dissociation curve, large incremental changes in PaO_2 produce little or no change in oxygen saturation.

Hazards

• None with the device itself
• Possible harm to the patient if readings are inaccurate

Maintenance

• Clean ear probe between patients.
• Calibrate device before each use.

TRANSCUTANEOUS OXYGEN AND CARBON DIOXIDE MONITORING

Description

Transcutaneous monitors allow the clinician to continuously monitor the patient's oxygenation or ventilation state. A modified Clark (for oxygen) and Severinghaus (for carbon dioxide) electrode employs a heating element attached to the patient's skin. Perfusion, blood pressure, skin thickness, and subcutaneous fat deposits affect accurate monitoring.

Objective

To monitor carbon dioxide and oxygen using a noninvasive technique.

Procedure

1. Ensure correct operation of transcutaneous unit by performing calibration procedure.
2. Approach the patient and explain the procedure.

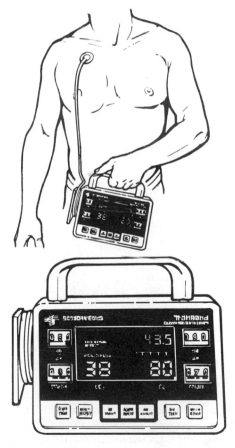

FIG. 7-17. *Transcutaneous O_2 and CO_2 monitor*

3. Select site for sensor placement. Upper chest and abdomen are good sites in infants as well as adults. Inner aspect of the arm and thigh may also give good correlation.
4. Prepare the skin site by rubbing area with isopropyl alcohol.
5. Apply one drop of electrolyte solution.
6. Apply the skin sensor on the drop of electrolyte.
7. Wait for stabilization to occur in approximately 10 minutes or less in neonates. Adults may take longer. Make sure your results are accurate. Compare results to a simultaneously obtained blood gas. Oxygen and carbon dioxide values will trend.
8. Set upper and lower alarm limits.
9. Change the sensor site every 2 to 6 hours.

Special Considerations

- Sensor temperature should not be changed after unit is attached to the patient.
- Inaccurate readings may occur if sensor is placed over bony areas.
- The longer the sensor is left in one position, the greater the chance of burn.
- Membranes should be reloaded at least every seven days.

Hazards

- Burns when sensor is left in one place too long or sensor temperature is too high
- Inaccurate estimation of arterial blood gas values

Maintenance

- Change sensor site every 2 to 6 hours.
- Initialize system with barometric pressure, site time, and patient temperature.
- Inspect membrane for visible damage. Note any sags, wrinkles, rips, or abrasions. Remembrane when damage is apparent or calibration fails. Membranes that are in use on a daily basis will usually last from 7 to 10 days when undamaged.

• Set sensor temperature:
  Adults 43.5°C
  Neonates 43.0°C
• Periodically remove the silver chloride that accumulates
  on the electrode. Follow manufacturer's instructions.

ARTERIAL PUNCTURE

Description

Arterial puncture is the method by which an arterial sample is obtained.

Objective

To obtain arterial blood for blood gas analysis.

Procedure

1. Assemble equipment necessary for arterial puncture:
   glass or plastic syringe with free-flowing barrel, prep

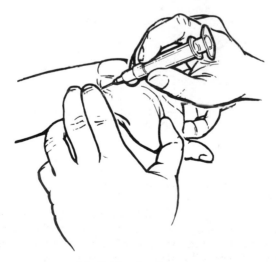

FIG. 7-18. *Arterial puncture*

pads, sterile gauze, sodium heparin, cork or rubber
stopper, clear hub, short bevel needles (#20–#25
gauge), container with ice, label, or prepackaged kits
with necessary components.

2. Approach the patient and explain the procedure.

INTERPRETATION OF ACID-BASE STATUS

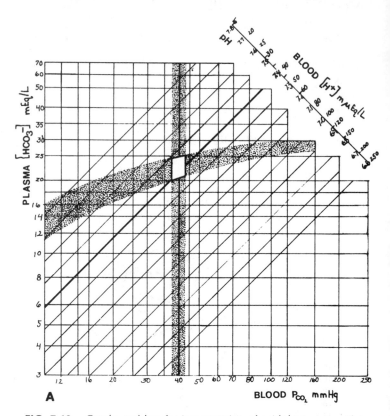

FIG. 7-19. *Graphs and key for interpretation of acid–base status. Plot
Pa_{CO_2} and pH points on graph A. The interpretation point is the intersection of these 2 points. Find that point on graph B. Read the corresponding
number and find its interpretation in C. To find plasma $[HCO_3^-]$, locate
Pa_{CO_2} and pH on A. From that point, draw a line parallel to the Pa_{CO_2} axis.
The intersection of this line with the $[HCO_3^-]$ axis indicates $[HCO_3^-]$
value. Note: pH falls 0.015 for each °C patient temperature rise. (Courtesy
of John Mathoefer, M.D.)*

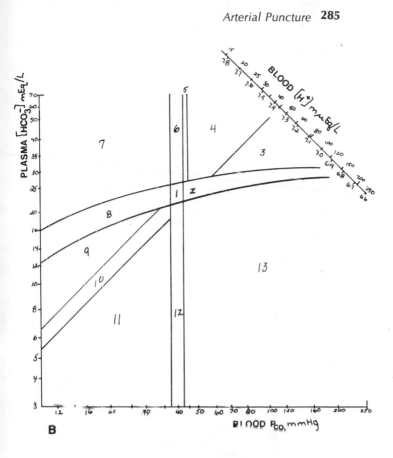

B

INTERPRETATION

1. Normal
2. Respiratory acidosis
3. Respiratory acidosis — compensated
4. Respiratory acidosis & metabolic alkalosis
5. Metabolic alkalosis — compensated
6. Metabolic alkalosis
7. Respiratory alkalosis & metabolic alkalosis
8. Respiratory alkalosis
9. Respiratory alkalosis — compensated
10. Metabolic acidosis & respiratory alkalosis
11. Metabolic acidosis — compensated
12. Metabolic acidosis
13. Metabolic acidosis & respiratory acidosis

C

3. Carefully select the puncture site.

- Prior to all radial punctures, perform an Allen's test to ensure collateral circulation.
- Locate both the ulnar and radial arteries.
- Clench hand into a fist; do this passively for neonates and infants.
- Compress both radial and ulnar arteries.
- Open hand completely.
- Release pressure on ulnar artery.
- If hand flushes upon release of ulnar artery, adequate collateral circulation exists.
- If poor or no flushing exists, do not use this site for puncture.

4. Prepare the syringe.

- Heparinize syringe and needle.
- Remove air from syringe.
- Replace cap on needle.

5. Prepare the puncture area and your own fingers with prep pads.
6. Palpate the puncture site very carefully, using a two-finger method.
7. Penetrate the artery with the needle at a 45 degree angle with the bevel facing the flow of blood.
8. Watch for a flash of blood into the hub of the needle.
9. Hold the needle inside the artery until the syringe fills to the desired level or aspirate the syringe to desired level if not self-filling.
10. Apply firm pressure with sterile gauze, remove needle from artery, and continue to maintain pressure for 5 minutes.
11. Remove any air bubbles from the syringe.
12. Stick the end of the syringe into stopper immediately.
13. Mix sample well.
14. Label syringe with patient's name, date, and time.
15. Place syringe in ice water bath.
16. Analyze immediately.

Special Considerations

- The radial artery is the artery of choice, followed by the brachial and femoral.

TABLE 7-9. OXYGENATION FORMULAS

	ABBREVIATION	FORMULA	RANGE	NORMAL
FIO_2	Fractional concentration of inspired oxygen		0.21–1	
PB	Barometric pressure		730–770 mm Hg*	
RQ	Respiratory quotient		0.69–1.1	.83
$PaCO_2$	Partial pressure of arterial carbon dioxide		20–80 mm H₂O*	35–45 mm Hg
PaO_2	Partial pressure of arterial oxygen		0–700 mm H₂O	70–100 mm Hg
PAO_2	Partial pressure of alveolar oxygen	$PAO_2 = PIO_2 - PaCO_2\left[FIO_2 + \left(\dfrac{1 - FIO_2}{RQ}\right)\right]$ $= [(P_B - PIH_2O)FIO_2]$ PIO_2 = partial pressure of oxygen in inspired gas (mm Hg) $PaCO_2$ = partial pressure of carbon dioxide in alveolar gas (often assumed to be equal to arterial carbon dioxide tension $PaCO_2$) FIO_2 = fraction of oxygen in inspired gas RQ = respiratory quotient	100–760 mm Hg	102 mm Hg

(Continued)

287

TABLE 7-9. OXYGENATION FORMULAS (Continued)

ABBREVIATION		FORMULA	RANGE	NORMAL
$P_{(A - a)}O_2$	Alveolar to arterial oxygen gradient	$P_{(A - a)}O_2 = P_1O_2 - P_ACO_2\left[F_1O_2 + \left(\dfrac{1 - F_1O_2}{RQ}\right)\right] - PaO_2$	30–50 mm Hg	30–50 mm Hg
$\dot{Q}_S/\dot{Q}_T$	Venous to arterial shunt	$\dfrac{\dot{Q}_S}{\dot{Q}_T} = \dfrac{(P_AO_2 - PaO_2)0.0031}{C(a - \bar{v})O_2 + P_AO_2 - PaO_2)(0.0031)}$	.01–.10*	.02–.05
		$\dot{Q}_S$ = shunted portion of cardiac output		
		$\dot{Q}_T$ = total cardiac output (lpm)		
		P_AO_2 = partial pressure of oxygen in alveolar gas (mm Hg)		
		PaO_2 = partial pressure of arterial oxygen (mm Hg)		
		$C(a - \bar{v})O_2$ = arteriovenous oxygen content difference (assumed to be 3.5 vol %)		
PaO_2/F_1O_2	Arterial to inspired oxygen gradient	$PaO_2/F_1O_2 = PaO_2/F_1O_2$	350–500 mm Hg	
		PaO_2 = partial pressure of arterial oxygen (mm Hg)		
		F_1O_2 = fractional concentration of inspired oxygen		

PaO_2/P_AO_2	Arterial to alveolar tension ratio	$PaO_2/P_AO_2 = \dfrac{PaO_2}{P_I - P_ACO_2}\left[FiO_2 + \left(\dfrac{1 - FiO_2}{RQ}\right)\right]$	0–1	.74–.82
Hgb	Hemoglobin		3–19 g	11–15 g
SaO_2	Arterial oxygen saturation		.7–1 (70–100%)*	.9–.99 (90%–99%)
SvO_2	Venous oxygen saturation		.5–.8 (50–80%)*	
PvO_2	Partial pressure of venous oxygen		15–50 mm Hg	45 mm Hg
CO	Cardiac output			
P_AO_2 required		$P_AO_2\text{ required} = \dfrac{PaO_2\text{ desired}}{\text{a/A }O_2\text{ calculated}}$	1–8.5 liter	5–6 liter
Desired FiO_2		$P_AO_2 = PIO_2 - (PaCO_2 \times 1.25)$ $P_AO_2 = (P_B - P_{H_2O})FiO_2 - (PaCO_2 \times 1.25)$ (stop at 100%)		

* On constant flow generator

- Always check for collateral circulation with radial artery.
- Compress the artery for at least 5 minutes following the puncture.
- Sample should be analyzed within 20 minutes.
- For patients on anticoagulant therapy with a history of bleeding disorder, decreased platelet count, or thrombolytic therapy, compression of the artery may be needed for an extended period of time.
- For patients with arteriosclerotic disease, compress artery only until bleeding stops.

Hazards

- Bleeding for patient on anticoagulant therapy or with history of bleeding
- Hematoma
- Nerve spasm
- Severing of the artery
- Arteriospasm
- Infection
- Thrombosis
- Loss of limb
- Spread of disease or infection if another person is stuck with the contaminated needle from an ill patient

Maintenance

- Examine the artery 5 minutes and 10 minutes after puncture to check for bleeding and complications.
- Dispose of blood gas kit properly.

REFERENCE

1. Banner MJ, Gallasher TJ, Bluth LI: A new microprocessor device for mean airway pressure measurement. Crit Care Med 9, No. 1: 51–53, 1981

BIBLIOGRAPHY

Askanazi J, Weissman C, Rosenbaum SH et al: Nutrition and the respiratory system. Crit Care Med 10, No. 3: 163–172, 1982

Burton GG, Hodgkin JE (eds): Respiratory Care: A Guide to Clinical Practice. Philadelphia, JB Lippincott, 1984

Grossman G: Nutritional assessment of critically ill patients. Resp Care 23: 856, 1978

Hess D, Good C, Didyoung R et al: The validity of assessing arterial blood gases 10 minutes after FiO_2 change in mechanically ventilated patients without chronic pulmonary disease. Resp Care 30, No. 12: 1037–1041, 1985

Levesque PR, Rosenberg H: Rapid bedside estimation of wasted ventilation (Vd/Vt). Anesthesiology 42, No. 1, 1975

Mathews P, Neubert D, Conover S, Dion B: Arterial blood gas equilibration time following changes in ventilator settings. Resp Ther 15, No. 6: 12–19, 1985

Popovich J, Bone RC, Wilson FJ, Hiller FC: Respiratory mass spectrometry. Resp Ther 10, No. 2, 1980

Reedinger M, Shellock F, and Swan HJC: Reading pulmonary artery and pulmonary capillary wedge pressure waveforms with respiratory variations. Heart Lung 10, No. 4: 675–678, 1981

Schroeder J, Daily E: Techniques in Bedside Hemodynamic Monitoring. St Louis, CV Mosby, 1981

Schweiss JF (ed): Continuous Measurement of Blood Oxygen Saturation in the High Risk Patient. San Diego, Beach International, 1983

Shapiro BA, Harrison RA, Walton JR: Clinical Application of Blood Gases. Chicago, Year Book Medical Pub, 1980

Spearman CB, Sheldon RL (eds): Egans Fundamentals of Respiratory Therapy, 4th ed. St Louis, CV Mosby, 1982

Trueblood DM: Development and Testing of a Gas Monitoring System for Measurement of Cutaneous PCO_2 and PO_2 in Neonates and Adults. Sensormedics Reprint 027

Wernerus H, Silva G, Wanner A: Accuracy of Drager & Wright ventilation meters. Resp Care 23: 856, 1978

infection control
Diane Blodgett

This chapter deals with the procedures for infection control, cleaning and decontamination, and bacteriological surveillance of respiratory therapy equipment. If we perform all the other elements of respiratory care correctly and neglect the infection control measures and the bacteriological monitoring of our equipment, we perform our duties for naught.

For respiratory therapy personnel, infection control measures should include aseptic handwashing procedures, aseptic handling of supplies and equipment, and strict adherence to the principles of isolation. This chapter includes all of these procedures.

Respiratory therapy equipment can provide a primary source of nosocomial infections. Therefore, infection control measures for equipment should include the use of filters and disposables, where appropriate, and the decontamination or sterilization of all permanent equipment.

The various methods of cleaning and decontamination of respiratory therapy equipment are summarized here in a comparison chart (Table 8-1). Different methods produce varying results; cleaning merely removes organic or inorganic material, while decontamination removes all pathogens. Sterilization means destruction of all microorganisms.

Whatever process you follow, adhere to certain guidelines. Keep dirty equipment in one area, clean in another. The process should flow from dirty (contaminated) to clean (decontaminated). The surfaces of large pieces of equipment should be cleaned, then wiped down with a decontaminating agent and labeled. When the decontamination process for smaller items is complete, the package label should include information on the type of process used, the initials of the therapist processing the equipment, the date of the processing, and the date of expiration. This information allows the equipment to be traced if you encounter a problem.

Monitoring your methods of decontamination or sterilization not only assures quality control, but also provides you with some reassurance that you are protecting the patient. Test the effluent gas since this gas comes in contact with the patient. However, rinse sampling may be appropriate in some cases. Test equipment in use to evaluate policies relating to length of equipment use. To double-check your method of surveillance and your decontamination or sterilization procedures, periodically contaminate a piece of equipment, take a bacteriological sample, process the equipment, and take another sample. Periodic culturing of stocked equipment helps to evaluate the appropriateness of policies for storage and shelf life. Keeping track of nosocomial respiratory infection also indicates whether overall policies work. Any changes in the incidence of hospital-acquired respiratory infections warrant examination.

ETHYLENE OXIDE STERILIZATION

Description

Ethylene oxide (ETO) sterilization brings about the destruction of microorganisms by the use of ETO gas at a certain relative humidity (50%), temperature (120°–135°F), concentration (12%), vacuum (25–27 inches), and time (3–4 hours). The microorganisms are killed by preventing their reproduction.

Objective

To kill all microorganisms present on equipment that is heat- or moisture-sensitive (*e.g.*, plastics, rubber, respirators).

(*Text continues on p. 296.*)

TABLE 8-1. METHODS OF CLEANING AND DECONTAMINATION

METHOD	CHARACTERISTICS OF PROCESS	ADVANTAGES	DISADVANTAGES	EQUIPMENT TO BE DECONTAMINATED
Dry heat (sterilization)	Very high temperatures Low moisture content	No toxic by-products Inexpensive	Damages heat-sensitive equipment Equipment cannot be identified through packaging. May have incomplete kill on short cycle	Equipment that cannot be disassembled
Steam autoclaving (sterilization)	High temperatures High moisture content High pressures	No toxic by-products. Completely kills all microorganisms including spores Inexpensive, fast	Damages heat and moisture-sensitive equipment. Equipment cannot be identified through some packaging	Surgical instruments Linen Some high density plastics
Ethylene oxide	Low temperature ETO and carrier gas (Freon) necessary Specific time, conc., tem., etc. must be adhered to	Completely kills all microorganisms Low temperature Visibility of equipment through plastic wrap	Expensive, time-consuming. Must completely dry and clean equipment first. Aeration necessary to remove toxic by-products Must have well-ventilated area	Plastics Rubber Respirators All items heat- or moisture-sensitive

Method	Mechanism	Advantages	Disadvantages	Materials
Chemical sterilization (decontamination or sterilization) Potentiated acid glutaraldehyde Aqueous buffered glutaraldehyde	Low pH liquid	Room temperature Lasts 4 weeks Fast; sterilizes in 1 hour at 60°C (10 minutes for disinfection)	Somewhat expensive, not appropriate for most electrical equipment. Can cause contact dermititis in users When equipment is improperly rinsed, toxic effect can result (burns). Possible recontamination during processing	Plastics Rubber Metal
Pasteurization (decontamination)	Hot water immersion	Relatively fast Easy No toxic by-products	Expensive initial outlay Recontamination can occur during processing. Not appropriate for electrical equipment or respirators Heat damage	Rubber Plastics Glass
Ultrasonic (decontamination)	Sound waves pass through fluid which vibrates; causing cleansing action	Fast Easy Uses water as fluid	Recontamination can occur during processing Expensive initial outlay	Rubber Plastics Surgical instruments Glass
Acetic acid (specific decontamination)	Low pH liquid	Inexpensive; for home use	Smell May be ineffective against most microorganisms	Home care equipment (better solutions are available)

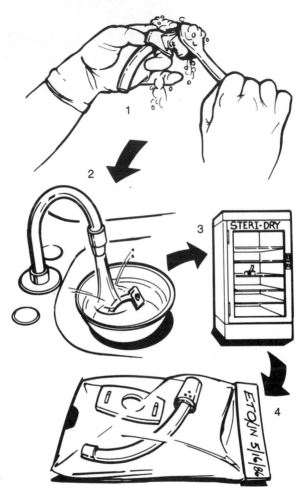

FIG. 8-1. *ETO sterilization*

Procedure

1. Disassemble equipment to be cleaned.
2. Clean equipment of all organic material.
3. Rinse equipment thoroughly to remove all cleaning residue.

4. Dry equipment completely.
5. Reassemble equipment in desired configuration.
6. Place equipment in plastic bag and insert indicator strip.
7. Remove as much air as possible from bag and seal bag with heat sealer, twist tie, or tape.
8. Place ETO tape on bag and mark package with date, expiration date, sterilization method, and technician's name.
9. Stack packages in ETO sterilizer chamber.
10. Follow manufacturer's instructions for ETO cycle.
11. When cycle is complete, remove from chamber and aerate either on shelf or in an aeration chamber.
12. Store in clean area.

Special Considerations

- Equipment must be clean and dry before being packaged.
- Complete aeration must be assured: 1 week on the shelf and 24 hours in aeration chamber.
- Plastic bags must be permeable to ETO.
- All sterilizing parameters (time, temperature, humidity, ETO concentration, and exposure time) must be met.
- Periodic microbiological sampling verifies effectiveness of process.

Hazards

- If equipment is not dry, water combines with ETO to form the toxic by-product ethylene glycol.
- Ethylene chlorohydrin, a toxic by-product, may be formed when rubber is processed.
- Because of the by-products, skin irritation, laryngeal edema, swelling, and burns may occur with improperly processed or aerated equipment.

Maintenance

- Shelf life for a tied or taped plastic package is 3 months; for a heat-sealed plastic package it is 1 year.

DRY HEAT STERILIZATION

Description

Dry heat autoclaving is a sterilization technique that brings about the destruction of microorganisms by very high

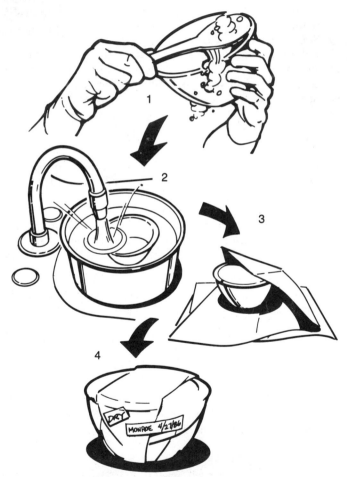

FIG. 8-2. *Dry heat sterilization*

temperatures over a long period of time (1–6 hours). The microorganisms are destroyed by the disruption of their cell membrane or coagulation of the protoplasm.

Objective

To kill all microorganisms present on equipment that can tolerate very high temperatures but cannot tolerate moisture (*e.g.,* moisture-sensitive equipment, equipment that cannot be disassembled).

Procedure

1. Disassemble equipment to be cleaned.
2. Clean equipment of all organic material.
3. Rinse equipment thoroughly to remove all cleanser residue.
4. Reassemble equipment in desired configuration.
5. Wrap equipment in porous towel or wrap.
6. Close wrap with indicator tape.
7. Wrap again with second towel or wrap unless a plastic/paper pouch is used.
8. Close wrap with indicator tape (heat-seal pouch, if used) and mark package with expiration date, sterilization method, and technician's name.
9. Stack packages in autoclave chamber.
10. Follow manufacturer's instructions for dry heat cycle.
11. Remove from chamber following completion of cycle.
12. Store in clean area.

Special Considerations

- Use where steam is unavailable.
- Plastics will melt.
- Do not use this method for electrical equipment.
- After processing, packs must remain dry to ensure sterility.
- Rubber may deteriorate.
- Periodic microbiological sampling verifies effectiveness of process.

Hazards

• Burns may occur with careless handling of packs.

Maintenance

• Shelf life for cloth or paper wrap is 30 days; for plastic/paper pouch it is 90 days.

COLD CHEMICAL STERILIZATION

Description

Cold chemical sterilization is a decontamination or sterilization technique that brings about the destruction of all microorganisms, including spores, in one hour (potentiated acid gluteraldehyde at 60°C) to ten hours (aqueous buffered gluteraldehyde); these two products are bactericidal in 10 to 20 minutes. This technique requires the immersion of the equipment in the sterilization liquid. Microorganisms are destroyed by protein denaturation or enzyme degradation.

Objective

To decontaminate or sterilize equipment that can tolerate immersion in a liquid at room temperature or slightly elevated temperatures (*e.g.,* plastics, rubber, metal).

Procedure

1. Disassemble the equipment to be cleaned.
2. Set aside equipment that cannot be immersed.
3. Clean equipment of all organic material.
4. Rinse equipment thoroughly to remove all cleanser residue.
5. Remove excess water.
6. Immerse equipment in sterilizing liquid for the required length of time (10–20 minutes for decontamination, 1–10 hours for sterilization). See Table 8-1.
7. Remove equipment from liquid.
8. Rinse thoroughly with sterile distilled water.

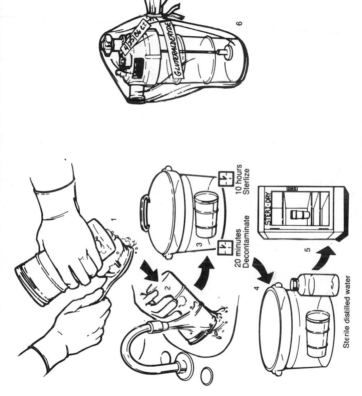

FIG. 8-3. Cold chemical sterilization

9. Dry completely in clean area.
10. Reassemble equipment.
11. Place equipment in plastic bag.
12. Seal bag with heat sealer, twist tie, or tape.
13. Mark package with date, expiration date, decontamination method, and technician's name.
14. Store in clean area.

Special Considerations

- Equipment must be clean before immersion in liquid.
- Completely immerse equipment in liquid; all surface areas must be in contact with liquid.
- To avoid a contact dermititis, use gloves when handling liquid.
- Rinse equipment completely before drying to remove toxic residue.
- Possible recontamination can occur during processing. Following processing, handle equipment with sterile technique.
- Equipment must be completely dry before repackaging.
- Verify effectiveness of process by periodic microbiological sampling.

Hazards

- Contact dermititis
- Recontamination following equipment removal from solution
- Toxic effects to patient when equipment is inadequately rinsed

Maintenance

- Shelf life of 3 months

STEAM AUTOCLAVE

Description

Steam autoclaving is a sterilization technique that brings about the destruction of microorganisms by steam under

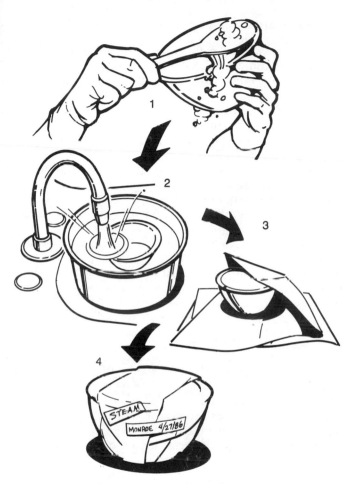

FIG. 8-4. *Steam autoclaving*

high temperature and pressure. The microorganisms are destroyed by the disruption of the cell membrane or the coagulation of the cell protoplasm.

Objective

To kill all microorganisms present on equipment that can tolerate moisture and high temperatures (*e.g.,* linen, surgical packs, utensils).

Procedure

1. Disassemble equipment to be cleaned.
2. Clean equipment of all organic material.
3. Rinse equipment thoroughly to remove all cleanser residue.
4. Reassemble equipment in desired configuration.
5. Wrap equipment in porous towel or steam wrap. Include sterilization indicator strip.
6. Close wrap with indicator tape.
7. Wrap again with second towel or wrap, unless plastic/paper pouch is used.
8. Close wrap with indicator tape (heat-seal pouch, if used) and mark with date, expiration date, sterilization method, and technician's name.
9. Stack packages to be steam autoclaved in steam chamber.
10. Follow manufacturer's instructions for steam cycle.
11. Remove from chamber following completion of cycle.
12. Store in clean area.

Special Considerations

- Electrical equipment can be harmed with this procedure.
- Plastics may melt.
- Rubber may deteriorate.
- Packs must remain dry to ensure sterility.
- Indicator tape will change from light to dark.
- Verify effectiveness of process by periodic microbiological sampling.

Hazards

- Burns may occur through careless handling of equipment.

Maintenance

- Shelf life for cloth wrap is 30 days, for paper wrap it is 30 to 60 days, and for plastic/paper pouch it is 90 days.

PASTEURIZATION

Description

Pasteurization is a decontamination technique that brings about the destruction of most microorganisms (except spores) by immersion of equipment in a hot (170°F) water

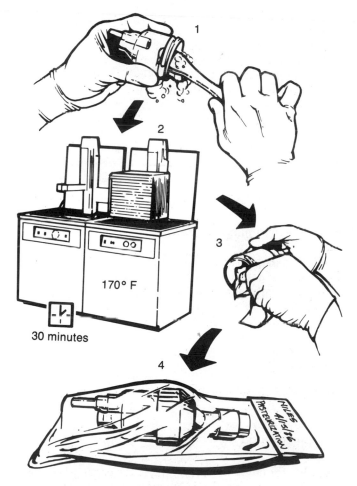

FIG. 8-5. *Pasteurization*

bath for one hour. The microorganisms are destroyed by the heat coagulation of the cell protoplasm.

Objective

To decontaminate equipment that can tolerate heat and immersion in a liquid (*e.g.,* plastics, rubber).

Procedure

1. Disassemble equipment.
2. Set aside equipment that cannot be immersed.
3. Clean equipment of all organic material.
4. Place equipment in a pasteurizing water bath.
5. Immerse equipment for one hour.
6. Remove equipment from water bath.
7. Dry completely in clean area.
8. Reassemble equipment.
9. Place equipment in plastic bag.
10. Seal bag with heat sealer, twist tie, or tape.
11. Mark package with date, expiration date, decontamination method, and technician's name.
12. Store in clean area.

Special Considerations

- Equipment must be clean before immersion in water bath.
- Equipment must be completely dry before packaging.
- Possible recontamination can occur during processing. Following processing, handle equipment with sterile technique.
- Verify effectiveness of process by periodic microbiological sampling.

Hazards

- Burns during processing
- Recontamination following removal from pasteurizer

Maintenance

- Shelf life of 3 months

ULTRASONIC CLEANER

Description

Ultrasonic cleaning is a decontamination technique that brings about the destruction of most microorganisms by the immersion of equipment in a liquid and the vibration of that liquid at a high frequency. The microorganisms are destroyed by disruption of cell membrane.

Objective

To decontaminate equipment that can tolerate immersion in a liquid at room temperature (*e.g.,* plastics, metal instruments).

Procedure

1. Disassemble equipment.
2. Set aside equipment that cannot be immersed.
3. Place equipment in ultrasonic cleaner.
4. Make sure distilled water covers equipment.
5. Add small amount of ultrasonic cleaner detergent.
6. Turn on ultrasonic cleaner.
7. Process equipment for 30 minutes.
8. Remove equipment from ultrasonic cleaner.
9. Dry completely in clean area.
10. Reassemble equipment.
11. Place equipment in plastic bag.
12. Seal bag with heat sealer, twist tie, or tape.
13. Mark package with date, expiration date, decontamination method, and technician's name.
14. Store in clean area.

Special Considerations

- Possible recontamination can occur during processing. Following processing, handle equipment with sterile technique.
- Equipment must be completely dry before packaging.
- Verify effectiveness of process by periodic microbiological sampling.

Hazards

• Recontamination

Maintenance

• Shelf life of 3 months

ACETIC ACID

Description

Acetic acid decontamination is the technique most often recommended to patients going home with respiratory therapy equipment. It involves the immersion of the equipment in a weak acetic acid solution.

Objective

To decontaminate home care equipment for the respiratory therapy patient.

Procedure

1. Disassemble equipment.
2. Clean equipment of all organic material.
3. Rinse thoroughly to remove all cleaner residue.
4. Immerse equipment in acetic acid solution (0.25%).
5. Let soak 20 minutes.
6. Remove equipment from acetic acid.
7. Rinse thoroughly. Remove water from tubing.
8. Drain-dry completely in clean area.
9. Reassemble equipment.
10. Place equipment in plastic bag.
11. Store in clean area.

Special Considerations

• This procedure should be used only for home care patients.
• The procedure should be done at the end of each day of therapy.
• Equipment may become recontaminated during processing.

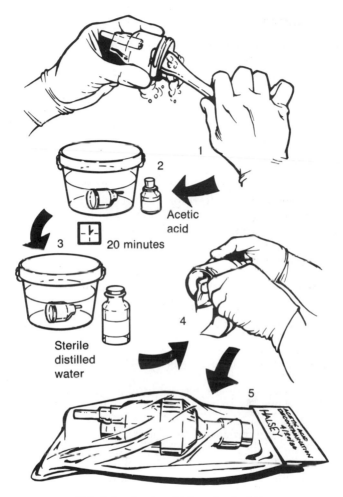

FIG. 8-6. *Acetic acid decontamination*

- Monitor patient infection rate. Rule out equipment as infection source.

Hazards

- Recontamination
- Lacks effectiveness against most bacteria

Maintenance

• New solution of acetic acid used each day
• Process equipment each day
• Shelf life of one day

BACTERIOLOGICAL SAMPLING OF EFFLUENT GAS

Description

This method of testing respiratory therapy equipment for possible contamination uses a direct sample of the effluent gas over or through bacteriologic media.

Objective

To detect contamination of aerosol or humidity-producing respiratory therapy equipment.

Procedure

1. Obtain sampling equipment (agar plates with sampling funnel attached).
2. Start humidity- or aerosol-producing device.
3. Set device so that the maximum aerosol is being produced.
4. Allow equipment to run for at least 10 seconds.
5. Remove lid from sampling plate.
6. Insert hose into diverting funnel.
7. Sample effluent gas for 10 seconds.
8. Remove tubing from funnel.
9. Remove funnel and replace lid on plate.
10. Mark plate with identification data.
11. Send culture to lab or incubate for 24 to 48 hours at 37°C.

Special Considerations

• Remove mouthpieces or adapters from respiration circuits before testing.

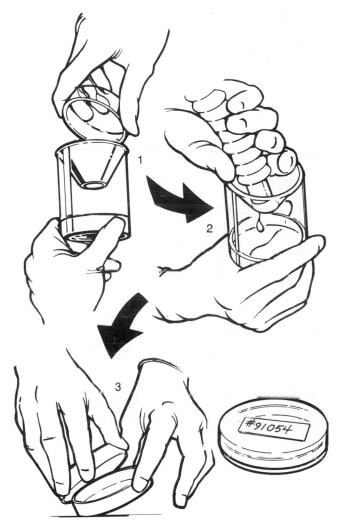

FIG. 8-7. *Bacteriological sampling of effluent gas*

- If more than 10 colonies are recovered, the level of contamination is unacceptable.
- Handle plates with care to avoid contamination.
- Mark each plate for positive identification.
- Refer to manufacturer's guidelines for flow and rate settings.

Hazards

- Spread of pathogenic organisms

Maintenance

- Commercial samplers may become outdated.

BACTERIOLOGICAL SAMPLING BY BROTH-RINSE METHOD

Description

This method of testing respiratory therapy equipment for possible contamination uses a bacteriologic broth which rinses through the equipment.

Objective

To detect contamination of respiratory therapy equipment.

Procedure

1. Obtain sampling equipment (nutrient broth, filter, sterile tube or flask, clamps).
2. For tubing: While holding tubing at each end, rinse some of broth through by raising and lowering each end alternately 50 times. For containers: Add rinse broth to container, close off opening, and shake vigorously for at least 30 seconds.
3. Filter broth into sterile tube or flask.
4. Mark tube or flask with identification data.

5. Send culture to lab or incubate for 24 to 48 hours at 37°C.

Special Considerations

• Handle samples with care to avoid contamination.
• Clamps can be used to seal end of flexible tubing.
• Small containers may be immersed in broth, which is then cultured.
• Mark each sample for positive identification.
• If more than 10 colonies are recovered, the level of contamination is unacceptable.

Hazards

• Spread of pathogenic organisms

Maintenance

• Use only currently dated supplies.

HANDWASHING TECHNIQUE

Description

Between each patient contact, respiratory therapy personnel should use a handwashing technique that minimizes the harboring and transmission of microorganisms.

Objective

To remove contaminants from hands of personnel and thus prevent the possibility of cross-contamination.

Procedure

1. Approach the sink, keeping body away from it.
2. Turn on and adjust the water to a warm temperature.
3. Wet hands.
4. Apply cleaning agent.

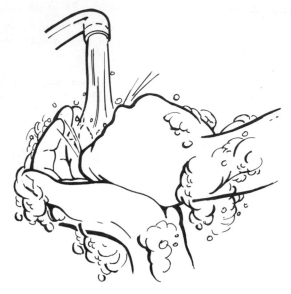

FIG. 8-8. *Handwashing*

5. Using vigorous movements, wash the hands for at least 30 seconds.
6. Rinse.
7. Repeat.
8. After the second washing, rinse well from the forearms down to the fingers.
9. Dry with paper towel.
10. Turn off water with second paper towel.

Special Considerations

• Remember to wash palms, between fingers, backs of hands, wrists, and forearms.
• Use a scrubbing, circular motion when washing.
• Any personnel with an open hand cut or wound should follow this technique and use gloves for each patient.

Hazards

• Spread of microorganisms if procedure is not followed carefully

Maintenance

• Use this procedure before and after each contact and for personal hygiene.

ASEPTIC TECHNIQUES

Description

Aseptic techniques are procedures or precautions that keep a person free from or prevent the entrance of pathogenic organisms.

Objective

To prevent the transmission of pathogens and protect the patient, the therapist, and others from infection.

Procedure

OPENING PACKAGES

1. Wash hands.
2. Open package away from you.
3. Whether package is single- or double-wrapped, touch only the outside.
4. Place package on flat surface.
5. The inside of the package is sterile.

POURING SOLUTIONS

1. Wash hands.
2. Pick up solution container and remove cap, placing it so that inside of cap is up.
3. Pour solution into sterile container. Do not touch container with bottle.
4. Throw remainder of solution away if single use. If multiple-use container, replace cap and mark the container with date and time.

Special Considerations

• If in doubt about the sterility of an item, consider it unsterile.

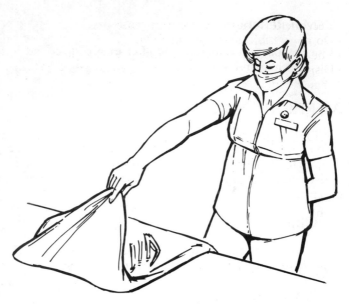

FIG. 8-9. *Aseptic technique for opening packages*

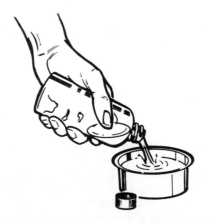

FIG. 8-10. *Aseptic technique for pouring solutions*

• Keep sterile items separate from unsterile.
• Do not reach across a sterile field.
• The edges of all items are considered unsterile.
• Dispose of the contents of solution bottles every 24 hours or more often.

Hazards

• Contamination of supplies during preparation or use

Maintenance

• Check dates of all supplies.
• Reprocess those supplies that become outdated.

ISOLATION TECHNIQUES

Description

Isolation techniques separate (set apart) the patient who has an infection from other patients and staff or protect the patient who is highly susceptible to infection.

Objectives

To prevent the spread of infection; to prevent cross-contamination.

Procedure

See Table 8-2.

Special Considerations

• When an infection is suspected, isolation techniques should be instituted. Cultures should confirm the infection.
• The type of isolation should be posted on the entrance to the room.

TABLE 8-2. ISOLATION PRECAUTIONS

TYPE OF ISOLATION	MASK	BEFORE AND AFTER CONTACT HAND-WASHING	CLOSED DOOR	DOUBLE-BAGGED TISSUES	DOUBLE-BAGGED RT EQUIPMENT	GOWNS	GLOVES
Wound & Skin		X		X			X
Enteric		X		X			X
Respiratory	X	X	X	X	X		
Strict	X	X	X	X	X	X	X
Protective	X	X	X			X	X

• These are not the only precautions necessary for isolation, but they represent the ones that respiratory therapy personnel will most likely follow.

Hazards

• If all precautions are not followed, the infection may be transmitted.

Maintenance

• Keep the patient in isolation until cultures are negative, drainage has stopped, or the patient's ability to fight infection has improved (protective isolation).

RESPIRATORY FILTERS

Description

Respiratory filters are devices that remove microorganisms from the air. Filters are used both internally and externally on respiratory therapy equipment.

Objective

To remove microorganisms from the air used to power respiratory therapy equipment and from the air directed to the patient from respiratory therapy equipment. To prevent cross-contamination from RT equipment. Filters may be used on the inspiratory or expiratory limb of a system.

Procedure

1. Check flow direction of filter.
2. Place external filters before the humidifier in line on main flow tubing.
3. Place external filter on supply line before the nebulizer.
4. Check resistance to air flow.
   a. Turn flow of respirator to 20 LPM.
   b. Disconnect tubing from both ends of filter.

c. Cycle respirator to inspiration.
d. Observe system pressure.
e. Connect filter to machine outlet. Do not connect respirator tubing.
f. Cycle respirator to inspiration.
g. Observe system pressure.
h. Difference should be less than 4 cm H_2O.

Special Considerations

• Do not allow filters to become wet or clogged.
• Replace when recommended (see Maintenance).

Hazards

• Diminished air flow with obstructed filter
• Loss of effectiveness when filter is used longer than recommended

Maintenance

• Use expiratory filters when appropriate.
• Use single-use filters only for one patient.
• Replace permanent filters every 5000 hours, or when resistance in filter has increased (4 cm H_2O).
• Replace internal filters at least every six months.
• Permanent filters should be steam autoclaved.

BIBLIOGRAPHY

Administrative standards for respiratory care services and personnel: An official statement from the American Association for Respiratory Therapy. Resp Care 28, No. 8: 1033–1038, 1983

Dixon RE (ed): Isolation Techniques for Use in Hospitals, 2nd ed. Washington, DC, Public Health Service, US Dept of HEW, 1975

Lennette EH, Spaulding EH, Truant JP: Manual of Clinical Microbiology. Washington, DC, American Society for Microbiology, 1974

Paluch, Bernard: Infection control and ventilator circuits. Resp Care 29, No. 9: 944, 1984

Wood LA, Rambo B: Nursing Skills for Allied Health Personnel, Vol 1, 2, and 3. Philadelphia, WB Saunders, 1977

ATI BOOKLETS

Principles and Practice of Autoclave Sterilization, Principals and Practice of Ethylene Oxide Sterilization. North Hollywood, Aseptic Thermo Indicator Co

appendices

MEASUREMENT CONVERSION FACTORS

Centimeter = inches × 2.54
Inch = centimeter/2.54
Meter = 39.37 inches

Units of Length

	MILLIMETERS	CENTIMETERS	INCHES	FEET	YARDS	METERS
1 mm	1.0	0.1	0.03937	0.00328	0.0011	0.001
1 cm	10.0	1.0	0.3937	0.03281	0.0109	0.01
1 in	25.4	2.54	1.0	0.0833	0.0278	0.0254
1 ft	304.8	30.48	12.0	1.0	0.333	0.3048
1 yd	914.40	91.44	36	3.0	1.0	0.9144
1 m	1000.0	100.0	39.37	3.2808	1.0936	1.0

Units of Weight

	GRAINS	GRAMS	APOTHECARIES OZ	AVOIRDUPOIS LB	KILOGRAMS
1 gr	1.0	0.0648	0.00208	0.0001429	0.000065
1 g	15.432	1.0	0.03215	0.002205	0.001
1 oz	480.0	31.1	1.0	0.06855	0.0311
1 lb	7000.0	453.5924	14.583	1.0	0.45354
1 kg	15432.358	1000.0	32.15	2.2046	1.0

Kilogram = pound × 2.2
Pound = kilogram/2.2

Units of Volume (Fluid or Liquid)

	MILLIMETERS	US DRAMS	INCHES³	US OZ	US QT	LITERS
1 ml	1.0	0.2705	0.061	0.03381	0.00106	0.001
1 fl dr	3.697	1.0	0.226	0.125	0.00391	0.00369
1 cu in	16.3866	4.4329	1.0	0.5541	0.0173	0.01639
1 fl oz	29.573	8.0	1.8047	1.0	0.03125	0.02957
1 qt	946.332	256.0	57.75	32.0	1.0	0.9463
1 liter	1000.0	270.52	61.025	33.815	1.0567	1.0

VOLUME (AIR OR GAS) CONVERSION FACTORS

1 Cubic centimeter = 0.06102 inch
1 Cubic meter = 35.314 cubic feet
1 Cubic meter = 1.3079 cubic yard
1 Cubic inch = 16.3872 cubic centimeters
1 Cubic foot = 0.02832 cubic meter

TEMPERATURE CONVERSION FACTORS

Centigrade = 5/9 Fahrenheit − 32
Fahrenheit = 9/5 Centigrade + 32

CLINICAL RANGE—TEMPERATURE CONVERSION

CENTIGRADE	FAHRENHEIT
36.0	96.8
36.5	97.7
37.0	98.6
37.5	99.5
38.0	100.4
38.5	101.3
39.0	102.2
39.5	103.1
40.0	104.0
40.5	104.9
41.0	105.8
41.5	106.7
42.0	107.6

FLOW RATE CONVERSION

Cubic feet/hour = cc/min × 0.00212
Cubic feet/hour = liters/min × 2.12
Liters/min = cubic feet/hour × 0.472

PRESSURE CONVERSION FACTORS

Lb/sq in = atmospheres × 14.696
Lb/sq in = inches of water × 0.3609
Lb/sq in = ft of water × 0.4335
Lb/sq in = in of mercury × 0.4912
Lb/sq in = kg/sq meter × 0.00142
Lb/sq ft = atmospheres × 2116.8
Lb/sq ft = in of water × 5.204
Lb/sq ft = feet of water × 62.48
Lb/sq ft = in of mercury × 79.727
Lb/cu in = gm/ml × 0.03613
Inches of water = inches of mercury × 13.60
Inches of water = cm of mercury × 5.3543
Ft of water = atmospheres × 33.95
Ft of water = inches of mercury × 1.133
Atmospheres = ft of water × 0.02947
Atmospheres = inches of mercury × 0.03342
Atmospheres = kg/sq cm × 0.9678
In of mercury = atmospheres × 29.921
In of mercury = lb/sq in × 2.036
Mm of mercury = atmospheres × 760.0
Kg/sq meter = lb/sq in × 703.1
Kg/sq meter = in of water × 25.40
Kg/sq meter = in of mercury × 345.32
Kg/sq meter = atmospheres × 10332.0

PRESSURE UNIT CONVERSIONS

TO CONVERT FROM	TO	MULTIPLY BY
cm H$_2$O	mm Hg	0.735
	inches Hg	0.0290
	psi	0.0142
mm Hg	cm H$_2$O	1.36
	inches Hg	0.0394
	psi	0.0193
inches Hg	mm Hg	25.4
	cm H$_2$O	34.5
	psi	0.491
psi	mm Hg	51.7
	cm H$_2$O	70.4
	inches Hg	2.04

☐ **Appendix B**
NORMAL AND ABNORMAL PATTERNS OF BREATHING

Apnea Cessation of ventilation in the resting expiratory position.

Apneusis Cessation of ventilation in the inspiratory position.

Apneustic breathing Apneusis interrupted periodically by expiration. May be rhythmic, *e.g.,* brain stem.

Breathing Alternating inspiration and expiration of air into and out of the lungs.

Breathing cycle From end expiration to end expiration.

Breathing frequency Number of breathing cycles per unit of time.

Breathing pattern Refers to the characteristics of the ventilatory activity.

Biots breathing Alternate hypernea (either tidal volume or frequency) and apnea occur in abrupt attacks for regular periods, *e.g.,* lesions of the medulla, meningitis.

Cheyne–Stokes breathing Pattern of breathing in which tidal volume first progressively increases and then progressively decreases, followed by a period of apnea; then the breathing sequence is repeated, *e.g.,* cardiac decompensation or cerebral terminal hypoxia.

Dyspnea Difficult or labored breathing, subjective feeling of shortness of breath.

Adapted from Slonin NB, Hamilton LH: Respiratory Physiology. St Louis, CV Mosby, 1981

Eupnea Normal spontaneous breathing.

Gasp A ventilatory movement consisting of a sudden brief inspiratory effort.

Hypernea Increased breathing, usually refers to increased tidal volume with or without increased frequency.

Hyperventilation Pulmonary ventilation exceeding the metabolic rate for respiratory gas exchange (P_aCO_2 less than normal values).

Hyponea Decreased breathing (either tidal volume or frequency).

Hypoventilation Pulmonary ventilation less than the metabolic rate for respiratory gas exchange (P_aCO_2 greater than normal values).

Kussmaul breathing Inspirations are forced and regular but expiration is unaffected, *e.g.,* diabetic acidosis.

Orthopnea Dyspnea that can be relieved by sitting in upright position.

Pant Rapid shallow breathing.

Respiration Gas exchange: *external*—between lungs and pulmonary circulation; *internal*—between arterial circulation system and the cell.

Tachypnea Increased frequency of breathing (polypnea).

Ventilation Volume of air that moved into and out of the lung per unit of time (minute volume = tidal volume × frequency).

□ Appendix C
COMMONLY USED ABBREVIATIONS

a arterial or artery

ac before meals

ad to; up to

ad lib as needed

amt amount

ant anterior

approx approximately (about)

AV atrioventricular

bid twice a day

BP blood pressure

BUN blood urea nitrogen

C Centigrade; Calorie; Celsius

c with
ca about
cap capsule
CBC complete blood count
cc cubic centimeters
CDC Center for Disease Control
cm centimeter
CNS central nervous system
CSF cerebrospinal fluid
CV cardiovascular
/d per day
D dose
DC discontinue
dil dilute
ECG (EKG) electrocardiogram (tracing of electrical heart activity)
EEG electroencephalogram (brain wave tracing)
ENT ear, nose, throat
ER emergency room
F Fahrenheit
f frequency
FDA Food and Drug Administration
fld fluid
GI gastrointestinal (stomach and intestine)
g gram
gr grain
gtt drop
h hour
Hgb hemoglobin
H₂O water
hs bedtime
I and O intake and output
IM intramuscular
IV intravenous (within vein)
kg kilogram
l liter
lab laboratory
lat lateral

lb pound
m meter
med medial
mEq milliequivalent
min minute
mg milligram
no number
noc night
NPO nothing by mouth
O₂ oxygen
OB obstetrics
OR operating room
os mouth
p pulse
Ped or Peds or Pedi pediatrics
po per os or by mouth
post-op postoperative (after surgery)
prn whenever necessary
pre-op preoperative (before surgery)
pt patient
PT physical therapy
Q2h every two hours
qd every day
qh every hour
qid four times a day
qod every other day
qs quantity sufficient
r or resp respirations
s without
Sol solution
stat at once
sup superior
T temperature
tab tablet
tid three times daily
TPR temperature; pulse, respirations
via by way of
wt weight

□ Appendix D
TERMS AND SYMBOLS USED IN RESPIRATORY PHYSIOLOGY

GENERAL

P Pressures in general

$\bar{X}$ Dash above any symbol indicates a mean value

$\dot{X}$ Dot above any symbol indicates a time derivative

$\ddot{X}$ Two dots above any symbol indicate the second time derivative

%X Per cent sign preceding a symbol indicates percentage of the predicted normal value

X/Y% Per cent sign *after* a symbol indicates a ratio function with the ratio expressed as a percentage. Both components of the ratio must be designated; e.g., $FEV_1/FEV\% = 100 \times FEV_1/FVC$

f Frequency of any event in time, e.g., respiratory frequency: the number of breathing cycles per unit of time

t Time

anat Anatomical

max Maximum

GAS PHASE SYMBOLS

Primary

V Gas volume in general. Pressure, temperature, and percent saturation with water vapor must be stated.

F Fractional concentration in dry gas phase

Qualifying

ɪ Inspired

ᴇ Expired

ᴀ Alveolar

ᴛ Tidal

ᴅ Dead space

ʙ Barometric

sᴛᴘᴅ Standard temperature and pressure, dry. These are the con-

Report from the ATS Pulmonary Nomenclature Subcommittee on Respiratory Physiology. ATS News, pp 12–15. Spring 1978

ditions of a volume of gas at O°C, at 760 torr, without water vapor

BTPS Body temperature (37°C), barometric pressure (at sea level = 760 torr), and saturated with water vapor

ATPD Ambient temperature, pressure, dry

ATPS Ambient temperature and pressure, saturated with water vapor

L Lung

BLOOD PHASE SYMBOLS

Primary

$\dot{Q}$ Volume flow of blood
C Concentration in blood phase
S Saturation in blood phase

Qualifying

b Blood in general
a Arterial. Exact location to be specified in text when term is used
v Venous. Exact location to be specified in text when term is used
v̄ Mixed venous
c Capillary. Exact location to be specified in text when term is used
c' Pulmonary end-capillary

PULMONARY FUNCTION

Lung Volumes (expressed as BTPS)

RV Residual volume: volume of air remaining in the lungs after maximum exhalation

ERV Expiratory reserve volume: maximum volume of air that can be exhaled from the end-tidal volume

VT Tidal volume: volume of gas that is inspired or expired during one ventilatory cycle

IRV Inspiratory reserve volume: maximum volume that can be inspired from an end-tidal inspiratory level

VL Volume of the lung, including the conducting airways. Conditions of measurement must be stated

IC Inspiratory capacity: volume that can be inspired from the end-tidal expiratory volume

IVC Inspiratory vital capacity: maximum volume measured on inspiration after a full expiration

VC Vital capacity: volume measured on complete expiration after the deepest inspiration, but without respect to the effort involved

FRC Functional residual capacity: volume of gas remaining in the lungs and airways at the end of a resting tidal expiration

TLC Total lung capacity: volume of gas in the lung and airways after as much gas as possible has been inhaled

RV/TLC% Residual volume to total lung capacity ratio, expressed as a per cent

V_D Physiological dead space: calculated volume (BPTS), which accounts for the difference between the pressures of CO_2 in expired gas and arterial blood. Physiological dead space reflects the combination of anatomical dead space and alveolar dead space, the volume of the latter increasing with the importance of the nonuniformity of the ventilation/perfusion ratio in the lung

$V_{D_{anat}}$ The alveolar dead-space volume (BTPS)

V_{D_A} The alveolar dead-space volume (BTPS)

Forced Respiratory Maneuvers (expressed as BTPS)

FVC Forced vital capacity: the volume of gas expired after full inspiration, and with expiration performed as rapidly and completely as possible

FIVC Forced inspiratory vital capacity: maximal volume of air inspired after a maximum expiration, and with inspiration performed as rapidly and completely as possible

FEV_t Denotes the volume of gas that is exhaled in a given time interval during the execution of a forced vital capacity

FEV_t/FVC% Ratio of timed forced expiratory volume to forced vital capacity, expressed as a percentage

PEF Peak expiratory flow (liters/min or liters/sec)

$\dot{V}max_{xx\%}$ Maximum expiratory flow (instantaneous) qualified by the volume at which measured, expressed as per cent of the FVC that has been exhaled. (Example: $\dot{V}max_{75\%}$ is the maximum expiratory flow after 75% of the FVC has been exhaled and 25% remains to be exhaled)

$\dot{V}max_{xx\%TLC}$ Maximum expiratory flow (instantaneous) qualified by the volume at which measured, expressed as per cent of the TLC that remains in the lung. (Example: $\dot{V}max_{40\%TLC}$ is the maximum expiratory flow when 40 per cent of the TLC remains in the lung)

FEF$_{x-y}$ Forced expiratory flow between two designated volume points in the FVC. These points may be designated as absolute volumes starting from the full inspiratory point or by designating the per cent of FVC exhaled

FEF$_{.2-1.2L}$ Forced expiratory flow between 200 ml and 1,200 ml of the FVC; formerly called maximum expiratory flow

FEF$_{25\%-75\%}$ Forced expiratory flow during the middle half of the FVC; formerly called maximum midexpiratory flow

MVV Maximum voluntary ventilation: maximum volume of air that can be breathed per min by a subject breathing quickly and as deeply as possible. The time of measurement of this tiring lung function test is usually between 12 and 30 sec, but the test result is given in liters (BTPS)/min

FET$_x$ Forced expiratory time required to exhale a specified FVC, e.g., FET$_{95\%}$ is the time required to deliver the first 95% of the FVC, FET$_{25\%-75\%}$ is the time required to deliver the middle half of the FVC

MIF$_x$ Maximum inspiratory flow (instantaneous). As in the case of the FET, appropriate modifiers designate the volume at which flow is being measured. Unless otherwise specified, the volume qualifiers indicate the volume inspired from RV at the point of measurement

Measurements of Ventilation

V̇E Expired volume per min (BTPS)

V̇I Inspired volume per min (BTPS)

V̇CO$_2$ Carbon dioxide production per min (STPD)

V̇O$_2$ Oxygen consumption per min (STPD)

R Respiratory exchange ratio in general. Quotient of the volume of CO_2 produced divided by the volume of O_2 consumed

V̇A Alveolar ventilation: physiological process by which alveolar gas is completely removed and replaced with fresh gas. The volume of alveolar gas actually expelled completely is equal to the tidal volume minus the volume of the dead space.

V̇D Ventilation per min of the physiologic dead space, BTPS

V̇D$_{anat}$ Ventilation per min of the anatomic dead space, that portion of the conducting airway in which no significant gas exchange occurs (BTPS)

V̇D$_A$ Ventilation of the alveolar dead space (BTPS), defined by the equation $\dot{V}_{D_A} = \dot{V}_D - \dot{V}_{D_{anat}}$

Mechanics of Breathing
(all pressures are expressed relative to ambient pressure unless otherwise specified)

Pressure Terms

Paw Pressure at any point along the airways

Pao Pressure at the airway opening, i.e., mouth, nose, tracheal cannula

Ppl Pleural pressure: the pressure between the visceral and parietal pleura relative to atmospheric pressure, in cm H_2O

Palv Alveolar pressure

PL Transpulmonary pressure: transpulmonary pressure, P_L = Palv − Ppl, measurement conditions to be defined

PstL Static recoil pressure of the lung; transpulmonary pressure measured under static conditions

Pbs Pressure at the body surface

Pes Esophageal pressure used to estimate Ppl

Pw Transthoracic pressure: pressure difference between parietal pleural surface and body surface. Transthoracic in the sense used means "across the wall." Pw = Ppl − Pbs

Ptm Transmural pressure pertaining to an airway or blood vessel

Prs Transrespiratory pressure: pressure across the respiratory system, Prs = Palv − Pbs = P_L + Pw

Flow–Pressure Relationships

R Flow resistance: the ratio of the flow-resistive components of pressure to simultaneous flow in cm H_2O/liter per sec

Raw Airway resistance calculated from pressure difference between airway opening (Pao) and alveoli (Palv) divided by the airflow, cm H_2O/liter/sec

RL Total pulmonary resistance includes the frictional resistance of the lungs and air passages. It equals the sum of airway resistance and lung tissue resistance. It is measured by relating flow-dependent transpulmonary pressure to airflow at the mouth

Rrs Total respiratory resistance includes the sum of airway resistance, lung tissue resistance, and chest wall resistance. It is measured by relating flow dependent transrespiratory pressure to airflow at the mouth

Rus Resistance of the airways on the upstream (alveolar) side of the point in the airways where intraluminal pressure equals Ppl (equal pressure point), measured during maximum expiratory flow

Rds Resistance of the airways on the downstream (mouth) side of the point in the airways where intraluminal pressure equals Ppl, measured during maximum expiratory flow

Gaw Airway conductance, reciprocal of Raw

Gaw/VL Specific conductance expressed per liter of lung volume at which Gaw is measured

Volume–Pressure Relationships

C Compliance: the slope of a static volume–pressure curve at a point, or the linear approximation of a nearly straight portion of such a curve expressed in liter/cm H_2O or ml/cm H_2O

Cdyn Dynamic compliance: the ratio of the tidal volume to the change in intrapleural pressure between the points of zero flow at the extremes of tidal volume in liter/cm H_2O or ml/cm H_2O

Cst Static compliance, value for compliance determined on the basis of measurements made during periods of cessation of airflow

C/VL Specific compliance: compliance divided by the lung volume at which it is determined, usually FRC

E Elastance: the reciprocal of compliance; expressed in cm H_2O/liter or cm H_2/ml

Pst Static components of pressure

W Work of breathing: the energy required for breathing movements

Diffusing Capacity

DL Diffusing capacity of the lung: Amount of gas (O_2, CO, CO_2) commonly expressed as ml gas (STPD) diffusing between alveolar gas and pulmonary capillary blood per torr mean gas pressure difference per min. Total resistance to diffusion for oxygen $\left(\dfrac{1}{D_{L_{O_2}}}\right)$ and CO $\left(\dfrac{1}{D_{L_{CO}}}\right)$ includes resistance to diffusion of the gas across the alveolar-capillary membrane, through plasma in the capillary, and across the red cell membrane ($1/D_M$), and the resistance to diffusion within the red cell arising from the chemical reaction between the gas and hemoglobin, ($1/\theta V_c$), according to the formulation $\dfrac{1}{D_L} = \dfrac{1}{D_M} + \dfrac{1}{\theta V_c}$

DM The diffusion capacity of the pulmonary membrane

θ The rate of gas uptake by 1 ml of normal whole blood per min for a partial pressure of 1 torr

Vc Average volume of blood in the capillary bed in milliliters

DL/VA Diffusion per unit of alveolar volume. DL is expressed STPD, and VA is expressed in liters (BTPS)

Respiratory Gases

Pa$_x$ Arterial tension of gas x, torr (mm Hg)

PA$_x$ Alveolar tension of gas x, torr (mm Hg)

Sa$_{O_2}$ Arterial oxygen saturation (per cent)

C Concentration: for example, Ca$_{CO_2}$ is the concentration of oxygen in a blood sample, including both oxygen combined with hemoglobin and physically dissolved oxygen, ordinarily expressed at ml O_2 (STPD)/100 ml blood, or mmole O_2/liter

PA − Pa Alveolar−arterial gas pressure difference: the difference in partial pressure of a gas (e.g., O_2 or N_2) in the alveolar gas spaces and that in the systemic arterial blood, measured in torr. For oxygen, as an example, PA$_{O_2}$ − Pa$_{O_2}$. Also symbolized AaD$_{O_2}$

Ca − Cv Arterial−venous concentration difference. For oxygen, as an example, Ca$_{O_2}$ − Cv$_{O_2}$

Pulmonary Shunts

Q̇s Shunt: vascular connection between circulatory pathways so that venous blood is diverted into vessels containing arterialized blood (right-to-left shunt, venous admixture) or vice versa (left-to-right shunt). Right-to-left shunt within the lung, heart, or large vessels due to malformations are more important in respiratory physiology. Flow from left to right through a shunt should be marked with a negative sign.

PULMONARY DYSFUNCTION

Altered Breathing

dyspnea An unpleasant *subjective* feeling of difficult or labored breathing

hyperventilation An alveolar ventilation that is excessive relative to the simultaneous metabolic rate. As a result the alveolar P_{CO_2} is significantly reduced below the normal for the altitude

hypoventilation An alveolar ventilation that is small relative to the simultaneous metabolic rate so that alveolar P_{CO_2} rises significantly above the normal for the altitude

Altered Blood Gases

hypoxia Any state in which the oxygen in the lung, blood, and/or tissues is abnormally low compared with that of normal resting person breathing air at sea level

hypoxemia A state in which the oxygen pressure and/or concentration in arterial blood is lower than its normal value at sea level. Normal oxygen pressures at sea level at 85–100 torr in arterial blood. In adult humans the normal oxygen concentration is 17–23 ml O_2/100 ml arterial blood

hypocapnia Any state in which the systemic arterial carbon dioxide pressure is significantly below 40 torr, as in hyperventilation

hypercapnia Any state in which the systemic arterial carbon dioxide pressure is significantly above 40 torr. May occur when alveolar ventilation is inadequate for a given metabolic rate (hypoventilation) or during CO_2 inhalation

Altered Acid–Base Balance

acidemia Any state of systemic arterial plasma in which the pH is significantly less than the normal value, 7.41 ± 0.02 in adult man at rest

alkalemia Any state of systemic arterial plasma in which the pH is significantly greater than the normal value, 7.41 ± 0.02 in adult man at rest

base excess (BE) Base excess: A measure of metabolic alkalosis or metabolic acidosis (negative values of base excess) expressed as the mEq of strong acid or strong alkali required to titrate a sample of 1 liter of blood to a pH of 7.40. The titration is made with the blood sample kept at 37°C, oxygenated, and equilibrated to P_{CO_2} of 40 torr

acidosis The result of any process that by itself adds excess CO_2 (respiratory acidosis) or nonvolatile acids (metabolic acidosis) to arterial blood. Acidemia does not necessarily result, because compensating mechanisms (increase of HCO_3 in respiratory acidosis, increase of ventilation and consequently, decrease of arterial CO_2 in metabolic acidosis) may intervene to restore plasma pH to normal

alkalosis The result of any process that, by itself, diminishes acids (respiratory alkalosis) or increases bases (metabolic alkalosis) in arterial blood. Alkalemia does not necessarily result, because compensating mechanisms may intervene to restore plasma pH to normal

Other

pulmonary insufficiency Altered function of the lung, which produces clinical symptoms that usually include dyspnea

acute respiratory failure Rapidly occurring hypoxemia, hypercarbia, or both caused by a disorder of the respiratory system. The duration of the illness and the values of arterial oxygen tension and arterial carbon dioxide tension used as criteria for this term should be given. The term acute ventilatory failure should be used only when the arterial carbon dioxide tension is increased. The term pulmonary failure has been used to indicate respiratory failure specifically caused by disorders of the lung

chronic respiratory failure Chronic hypoxemia or hypercapnia caused by a disorder of the respiratory system. The duration of the condition and the values of arterial oxygen tension and arterial carbon dioxide tension used as criteria for this term should be given

obstructive ventilatory defect Slowing of air flow during forced ventilatory maneuvers

restrictive ventilatory defect Reduction of vital capacity *not* explainable by airflow obstruction

impairment A measurable degree of anatomic or functional abnormality that may or may not have clinical significance. Permanent impairment is that which persists for some period of time, e.g., one year after maximum medical rehabilitation has been achieved

disability A legally or administratively determined state in which a patient's ability to engage in a specific activity under certain circumstances is reduced or absent because of physical or mental impairment. Other factors, such as age, education, and customary way of making a livelihood, are considered in evaluating disability. Permanent disability exists when no substantial improvement of the patient's ability to engage in the specific activity can be expected

REFERENCES

1. (Pappenheimer Committee) Standrdization of definitions and symbols in respiratory physiology. Fed Proc 9: 602, 1950
2. Glossary on respiration and gas exchange. J Appl Physiol 34: 549, 1973
3. Mead J, Milic-Emili J: Theory and methodology in respiratory mechanics with glossary of symbols. In Handbook of Physiology Respiration I, pp 363–364
4. Hyatt RE: Dynamic lung volumes. In Handbook of Physiology Respiration II, p 1386

5. Clinical spirometry (ACCP Committee). Chest 43: 214, 1963
6. Gandevia B, Hugh-Jones P: Terminology for measurements of ventilatory capacity: A report to the Thoracic Society. Thorax 12: 290, 1957
7. Pulmonary terms and symbols: A report of the ACCP-ATS Joint Committee on Pulmonary Nomenclature. Chest 67: 583, 1975

☐ Appendix E
NORMAL VITAL SIGNS

Pulse: Normal Values

Infants	112–130 beats/min
Adult	70–80 beats/min
Elderly	56–62 beats/min

Respiratory Rate: Normal Values

Infants	30–50 breaths/min
Adults	12–20 breaths/min

Blood Pressure: Normal Values

Infants	80/58–50/40
Adults	110/60–148/90

Temperature: Normal Values

Oral: 37°C or 98.6°F
Rectal: 37.3–37.6°C or 99.1–100.1°F

NORMAL BLOOD GAS VALUES

ARTERIAL	PREMATURE	TERM INFANT	CHILD	ADULT
pH	7.35–7.39	7.26–7.41	7.35–7.45	7.35–7.45
$PaCO_2$	38–44	34–54	35–45	35–45
PaO_2	65–80	60	75–100	75–100
O_2Sat	40–90%	40–95%	95–98%	95–98%
CO_2 Content	19–27 mEq/liter	20–26	18–27	24–30
BE	(−10)–(−2)	(−7)–(−1)	(−4)–(+2)	(+2)–(−2)
O_2 Content	15–23 vol%	(−1)–(−1)	(−4)–(+2)	(+2)–(−2)
O_2 Capacity	1.39 ml/g hemoglobin	(−1)–(−1)	(−4)–(+2)	(+2)–(−2)

☐ **Appendix F**
COMMONLY USED CRITICAL CARE FORMULAS

Body Surface Area

$$BSA = Wt^{0.425} \times Ht^{0.725} \times 0.007184 \qquad Wt = kg$$
(sq meters) (kg) (cm) $\qquad$ Ht = cm

Alveolar Air Equation: Alveolar − Arterial

$$P_AO_2 = (P_B - P_{H_2O})(F_IO_2) - \frac{(PaCO_2)}{.8}$$
Normal on Room Air: $P_B = 760$: 98–102

a/A Gradient

$$P(_A - _a)O_2 = P_AO_2 - PaO_2$$
Normal on Room Air: 10–15
Normal on Oxygen: 30–50

Shunt Equation

$$\frac{\dot{Q}s}{\dot{Q}t} = \frac{CcO_2 - CaO_2}{CcO_2 - C\bar{v}O_2} \qquad \text{Normal: } \leq 5\%$$

Systemic Vascular Resistance

$$SVR = \frac{MAP - CVP}{CO} \times 79.9 \text{ dyne/sec/cm}^{-5}$$
Normal: 800–1200

Pulmonary Vascular Resistance

$$PVR = \frac{MPAP - PWP}{CO} \times 79.9 \text{ dyne/sec/cm}^{-5}$$
Normal: 80–100

Arterial–Venous O_2 Content Difference

$$A{-}vO_2 = CaO_2 - C\bar{v}O_2 \quad \text{Normal: 3–15 Vol \%}$$

Anatomical Dead Space

$$V_D(anat) = V_T\left(1 - \frac{F_ECO_2}{F_ACO_2}\right) - \text{mechanical dead space}$$

Normal lcc/lb Ideal Body Weight

Ratio Dead Space to Tidal Volume

$$\frac{V_D}{V_T} = \frac{P_AO_2 - P_ECO_2}{P_AO_2}$$

or

$$\frac{V_D}{V_T} = \frac{PaCO_2 - P_ECO_2}{PaCO_2}$$

or

$$\frac{V_D}{V_T} = \frac{P_{ET}CO_2 - P_ECO_2}{P_{ET}CO_2}$$

Normal: .30–.35

Physiological Dead Space

$$V_D(phys) = V_T\left[\frac{1 - F_ECO_2(P_B - 47)}{PaCO_2}\right] - \text{mechanical dead space}$$

Oxygen Content

Capillary oxygen content

$$CcO_2 = (Hgb \times O_2Sat \times 1.39) + (0.003 \times P_AO_2)$$
$$(ScO_2) \quad \text{Normal: 9–10 Vol \%}$$

Arterial oxygen content

$$CaO_2 = (Hgb \times O_2Sat \times 1.39) + (PaO_2 \times 0.0031)$$
$$(SaO_2) \quad \text{Normal: 9–10 Vol \%}$$

Mixed venous oxygen content

$$C\bar{v}O_2 = (Hgb \times O_2Sat \times 1.39) + (P\bar{v}O_2 \times 0.0031)$$
$$(SvO_2) \quad \text{Normal: 4–6 Vol \%}$$

Mean Arterial Pressure

$$MAP = \frac{\text{systolic} - \text{diastolic}}{3} + \text{diastolic}$$

Normal: 75–90

Cardiac Output

$$\dot{Q} = \frac{\dot{V}CO_2}{(C\bar{v}CO_2 - CaCO_2)}$$

noninvasive

$$\dot{Q} = \frac{\dot{V}O_2}{CaO_2 - C\bar{v}O_2}$$

Fick equation
Normal: 4–6 liter/min

Cardiac Index

$$CI = \dot{Q}/BSA$$ Units: liter/min/m^2

O_2 Uptake

$$\dot{V}O_2 = \left[\dot{V}_E \times \frac{1 - F_EO_2 - FCO_2}{1 - F_IO_2 \quad F_ICO_2} \times F_IO_2 \right] - F_EO_2$$

Normal: 250 ml/liter/min

CO_2 Production

$$\dot{V}CO_2 - V_E \times (F_ECO_2 - F_ICO_2)$$

Normal: 200 ml/liter/min

RER (RQ)

$$R = \frac{\dot{V}CO_2}{\dot{V}O_2}$$ Normal = .8

Ventilatory Equivalents

Oxygen

$$V_EO_2 = \frac{\dot{V}_{E(BTPS)}}{\dot{V}O_{2(STPD)}}$$ Normal: 25 liters air
to consume 1 liter O_2

Carbon dioxide

$$V_ECO_2 = \frac{\dot{V}_{E(BTPS)}}{\dot{V}CO_{2(STPD)}}$$ Normal: 20 liters to
produce 1 liter CO_2

Compliance

$$C = \frac{\Delta V}{\Delta P}$$

Normal lung compliance: 100 ml/cm H_2O
Normal compliance of lung and chest wall in mechanically ventilated
patients: 70 ml/cm H_2O

Compliance: Dynamic

$$Cdyn = \frac{\Delta V}{\Delta P} \text{ (Peak Pressure)}$$
Normal: see above under Compliance

Compliance: Static

$$Cst = \frac{\Delta V}{\Delta P} \text{ (Plateau Pressure)} \qquad \text{Normal}$$

Compliance: Static (with PEEP)

$$Cst = \frac{\text{spirometer volume } - \text{ tube expansion volume}}{\text{plateau pressure } - \text{ PEEP}} \quad \text{Normal}$$

Airway Resistance

$$Raw = \frac{\text{Peak Pressure (Pp) } - \text{ static Pressure (Pst)}}{\dot{V}\text{(flow)}}$$
Normal: 2–3 cm H_2O/liter/s

Oxygen Delivery/Oxygen Transport

$$O_{2D} = \dot{Q}(CaO_2) \qquad \text{Normal}$$

□ **Appendix G**
LABORATORY TESTS—NORMAL VALUES

BLOOD, PLASMA OR SERUM VALUES

	REFERENCE RANGE	
DETERMINATION	**Conventional**	**SI**
Acetoacetate plus acetone	0.3–2.0 mg/100 ml	3–20 mg/l
Aldolase	1.3–8.2 mU/ml	12–75 nmol·s⁻¹l
Alpha amino nitrogen	3.0–5.5 mg/100 ml	2.1–3.9 mmol/l

Scully RE (ed): case records of the Massachusetts Genera Hospital. N Engl J Med 302: 37–48, 1980. Abbreviations used: SI, Système international d'Unités; d, 24 hours; P, plasma; S, serum; B, blood; U, urine; l, liter; h, hour; and s, second.

BLOOD, PLASMA OR SERUM VALUES *(Continued)*

	REFERENCE RANGE	
DETERMINATION	**Conventional**	*SI*
Ammonia	80–110 μg/100 ml	47–65 μmol/l
Amylase	4–25 U/ml	4–25 arb. unit
Ascorbic acid	0.4–1.5 mg/100 ml	23–85 μmol/l
Barbiturate	.0 Coma level: phenobarbital, approximately 10 mg/100 ml; most other drugs, 1–3 mg per 100 ml	0 μmol/l
Bilirubin (van den Bergh test)	One minute: 0.4 mg/100 ml	up to 7 μmol/l
	Direct: 0.4 mg/100 ml. Total: 1.0 mg/100 ml Indirect is total minus direct	up to 17 μmol/l
Blood volume	8.5–9.0% of body weight in kg	80–85 ml/kg
Bromide	0 Toxic level: 17 meq/l	0 mmol/l
Bromsulphalein (BSP)	Less than 5% retention	<0.05 l
Calcium	8.5–10.5 mg/100 ml (slightly higher in children)	2.1–2.6 mmol/l
Carbon dioxide content	24–30 meq/l 20–26 meq/l in infants (as HCO_3^-)	24–30 mmol/l
Carbon monoxide	Symptoms with over 20% saturation	0(1)
Carotenoids	0.8–4.0 μg/ml	1.5–7.4 μmol/l
Ceruloplasmin	27–37 mg/100 ml	1.8–2.5 μmol/l
Chloride	100–106 meq/l	100–106 mmol/l
Cholinesterase (pseudocholinesterase)	0.5 pH U or more/h 0.7 pH U or more/h for packed cells	0.5 or more arb. unit
Copper	Total: 100–200 μg/100 ml	16–31 μmol/l
Creatine phosphokinase (CPK)	Female 5–35 mU/ml Male 5–55 mU/ml	0.08–0.58 μmol · s^{-1}/l
Creatinine	0.6–1.5 mg/100 ml	60–130 μmol/l
Doriden (Glutethimide)	0 mg/100 ml	0 μmol/l
Ethanol	0.3–0.4%, marked intoxication; 0.4–0.5% alcoholic stupor; 0.5% or over, alcoholic coma	65–87 mmol/l 87–109 mmol/l >109 mmol/l
Glucose	Fasting: 70–110 mg/100 ml	3.9–5.6 mmol/l
Iron	50–150 μg/100 ml (higher in males)	9.0–26.9 μmol/l

(Continued)

BLOOD, PLASMA OR SERUM VALUES *(Continued)*

	REFERENCE RANGE	
DETERMINATION	**Conventional**	*SI*
Iron-binding capacity	250–410 µg/100 ml	44.8–73.4 µmol/l
Lactic acid	0.6–1.8 meq/l	0.6–1.8 mmol/l
Lactic dehydrogenase	60–120 U/ml	1.00–2.00 µmol · s⁻¹/l
Lead	50 µg/100 ml or less	up to 2.4 µmol/l
Lipase	2 U/ml or less	up to 2 arb. unit
Lipids		
Cholesterol	120–220 mg/100 ml	3.10–5.69 mmol/l
Cholesterol esters	60–75% of cholesterol	
Phospholipids	9–16 mg/100 ml as lipid phosphorus	2.9–5.2 mmol/l
Total fatty acids	190–420 mg/100 ml	1.9–4.2 g/l
Total lipids	450–1000 mg/100 ml	4.5–10.0 g/l
Triglycerides	40–150 mg/100 ml	0.4–1.5 g/l
Lipoprotein electro- phoresis (LEP)		
Lithium	Toxic level 2 meq/l	2 mmol/l
Magnesium	1.5–2.0 meq/l	0.8/1.3 mmol/l
Methanol	0	
5'Nucleotidase	0.3–3.2 Bodansky U	30–290 nmol · s⁻¹/l
Osmolality	285–295 mOsm/kg water	285–295 mmol/kg
Oxygen saturation (arterial)	96–100%	0.96–1.00 l
P$_{CO_2}$	35–45 mm Hg	4.7–6.0 kPa
pH	7.35–7.45	same
P$_{O_2}$	75–100 mm Hg (dependent on age) while breathing room air Above 500 mm Hg while on 100% O_2	10.0–13.3 kPa
Phenylalanine	0–2 mg/100 ml	0–120 µmol/l
Phenytoin (Dilantin)	Therapeutic level, 5–20 µg/ml	19.8–79.5 µmol/l
Phosphatase (acid)	Male—Total: 0.13–0.63 Sigma U/ml Female—Total: 0.01–0.56 Sigma U/ml Prostatic: 0–0.7 Fishman-Lerner U/100 ml	2.8–156 nmol · s⁻¹/l
Phosphatase (alkaline)	13–39 IU/l; infants and adolescents up to 104 IU/l	0.22–0.65 µmol · s⁻¹/l up to 1.26 µmol · s⁻¹/l
Phosphorus (inorganic)	3.0–4.5 mg/100 ml (infants in 1st year up to 6.0 mg/ 100 ml)	1.0–1.5 mmol/l
Potassium	3.5–5.0 meq/l	3.5–5.0 mmol/l

BLOOD, PLASMA OR SERUM VALUES *(Continued)*

	REFERENCE RANGE	
DETERMINATION	**Conventional**	*SI*
Primidone (Mysoline)	Therapeutic level 4–12 µg/ml	18–55 µmol/l
Protein: Total	6.0–8.4 g/100 ml	60–84 g/l
Albumin	3.5–5.0 g/100 ml	35–50 g/l
Globulin	2.3–3.5 g/100 ml	23–35 g/l
Electrophoresis	% of total protein	
Albumin	52–68	0.52–0.681
Globulin:		
Alpha$_1$	4.2–7.2	0.042–0.072/l
Alpha$_2$	6.8–12	0.068–0.12/l
Beta	9.3–15	0.093–0.15/l
Gamma	13–23	0.13–0.23/l
Pyruvic acid	0–0.11 meq/l	0–0.11 mmol/l
Quinidine	Therapeutic: 1.5–3 µg/ml	4.6–9.2 µmol/l
	Toxic: 5–6 µg/ml	15.4–18.5 µmol/l
Salicylate:	0	
Therapeutic	20–25 mg/100 ml;	1.4–1.8 mmol/l
	25–30 mg/100 ml to age 10 yrs. 3 h post dose	1.8–2.2 mmol/l
Toxic	Over 30 mg/100 ml; over 20 mg/100 ml after age 60	over 2.2 mmol/l over 1.4 mmol/l
Sodium	135–145 meq/l	135–145 mmol/l
Sulfate	0.5–1.5 mg/100 ml	0.05/1.2 mmol/l
Sulfonamide	0 mg/100 ml Therapeutic: 5–15 mg 100/ml	0 mmol/l
Thymol:		
Flocculation	Up to 1 + in 24 hr	up to 1 + arb. unit
Turbidity	0–4 U	0–4 arb. unit
Transaminase (SGOT) (aspartate amino-transferase)	10–40 U/ml	0.00–0.32 µmol · s^{-1}/l
Urea nitrogen (BUN)	8–25 mg/100 ml	2.9–8.9 mmol/l
Uric acid	3.0–7.0 mg/100 ml	0.18–0.42 mmol/l
Vitamin A	0.15–0.6 µg/ml	0.5–2.1 µmol/l
Vitamin A tolerance test	Rise to twice fasting level in 3 to 5 h.	

URINE VALUES

	REFERENCE RANGE	
DETERMINATION	**Conventional**	*SI*
Acetone plus acetoacetate (quantitative)	0	0 mg/l
Alpha amino nitrogen	64–199 mg/d; not over 1.5% of total nitrogen	4.6–14.2 mmol/d
Amylase	24–76 U/ml	24–76 arbitrary units
Calcium	150 mg/d or less	3.8 or less mmol/d
Catecholamines	Epinephrine: under 20 μg/d Norepinephrine: under 100 μg/d	<55 nmol/d <590 nmol/d
Chorionic gonadotropin	0	0 arb. unit
Copper	0–100 μg/d	0–1.6 μmol/d
Coproporphyrin	50–250 μg/d Children under 80 lb. 0–75 μg/d	80–380 nmol/d 0–115 nmol/d
Creatine	Under 100 mg/d or less than 6% of creatinine. In pregnancy: up to 12%. In children under 1 yr.: may equal creatinine. In older children: up to 30% of creatinine	<0.75 nmol/d
Creatinine	15–25 mg/kg or body weight/d	0.13–0.22 mmol $\cdot$ kg^{-1}/d
Creatinine clearance	150–180 l/d (104–125 ml/min) per 1.73 m^2 of body surface	1.7–2.1 ml/s
Cystine or cysteine	0	0
Follicle-stimulating hormone: Follicular phase Mid-cycle Luteal phase Menopausal Men	 5–20 IU/d 15–60 IU/d 5–15 IU/d 50–100 IU/d 5–25 IU/d	same
Hemoglobin and myoglobin	0	
Homogentisic acid	0	
5-Hydroxyindole acetic acid	2–9 mg/d (women lower than men)	10–45 μmol/d
Lead	0.08 μg/ml or 120 μg or less/d	0.39 μmol/l or less
Phenolsulfonphthalein (PSP)	At least 25% excreted by 15 min; 40% by 30 min; 60% by 120 min	0.25 l
Phenylpyruvic acid	0	0

URINE VALUES *(Continued)*

DETERMINATION	REFERENCE RANGE			
	Conventional		*SI*	
Phosphorus (inorganic)	Varies with intake; average 1 g/d		32 mmol/d	
Porphobilinogen	0		0	

Protein:
  Quantitative
  Electrophoresis
	<150 mg/24 h
	(see blood protein)
			<0.15 g/d	

Steroids:

	Age	*Male*	*Female*	*μmol/d*	*μmol/d*
17-Kerosteroids (per day)	10	1–4 mg	1–4 mg	3–14	3–14
	20	6–21	4–16	21–73	14–56
	30	8–26	4–14	28–90	14–49
	50	5–18	3–9	17–62	10–31
	70	2–10	1–7	7–35	3–24

DETERMINATION	Conventional	SI
17-Hydroxysteroids	3–8 mg/d (women lower than men)	8–22 μmol/d as hydrocortisone

Sugar:
  Quantitative glucose
  Identification of
    reducing sub-
    stances
	0	0 mmol/l

Fructose	0	0 mmol/l
Pentose	0	0 mmol/l
Titratable acidity	20–40 meq/d	20–40 mmol/d
Urobilinogen	Up to 1.0 Ehrlich U	to 1.0 arb. unit
Uroporphyrin	0	0 nmol/d
Vanillylmandelic acid (VMA)	Up to 9 mg/24 h	up to 45 μmol/d

SPECIAL ENDOCRINE TESTS: STEROID HORMONES

	REFERENCE RANGE	
DETERMINATION	***Conventional***	***SI***
Aldosterone	Excretion: 5–19 μg/24 hr	14–53 nmol/d
	Supine: 48 ± 29 pg/ml	133 ± 80 pmol/l
	Upright: (2 h) 65 ± 23 pg/ml	180 ± 64 pmol/l
	Supine: 107 ± 45 pg/ml	279 ± 125 pmol/l
	Upright: (2 h) 239 ± 123 pg/ml	663 ± 341 pmol/l
	Supine: 175 ± 75 pg/ml	485 ± 208 pmol/l
	Upright: (2 h) 531 ± 228 pg/ml	1476 ± 632 pmol/l
Cortisol	8 a.m.: 5–25 μg/100 ml	0.14–0.69 μmol/l
	8 p.m.: Below 10 μg/100 ml	0–0.28 μmol/l
	4 h ACTH test: 30–45 μg/100 ml	0.83–1.24 μmol/l
	Overnight suppression test: Below 5 μg/100 ml	<0.14 nmol/l
	Excretion: 20–70 μg/24 h	55–193 nmol/d
11-Deoxycortisol	Responsive: Over 7.5 μg/100 ml	>0.22 μmol/l
Testosterone	Adult male: 300–1100 ng/100 ml	10.4–38.1 nmol/l
	Adolescent male: Over 100 ng/100 ml	>3.5 nmol/l
	Female: 25–90 ng/100 ml	0.87–3.12 nmol/l
Unbound testosterone	Adult male: 3.06–24.0 ng/100 ml	106–832 pmol/l
	Adult female: 0.09–1.28 ng/100 ml	3.1–44.4 pmol/l

SPECIAL ENDOCRINE TESTS: POLYPEPTIDE HORMONES

	REFERENCE RANGE	
DETERMINATION	Conventional	SI
Adrenocorticotropin (ACTH)	15–70 pg/ml	3.3–15.4 pmol/l
Calcitonin	Undetectable in normals. >100 pg/ml in medullary carcinoma	0 >29.3 pmol/l
Growth hormone	Below 5 ng/ml Children: Over 10 ng/ml Male: Below 5 ng/ml Female: Up to 30 ng/ml Male: Below 5 ng/ml Female: Below 10 ng/ml	<233 pmol/l >465 pmol/l <233 pmol/l 0–1395 pmol/l <233 pmol/l 0–465 pmol/l
Insulin	6–26 μU/ml Below 20 μU/ml Up to 150 μU/ml	43–187 pmol/l <144 pmol/l 0–1078 pmol/l
Luteinizing hormone	Male: 6–18 mU/ml Female: 5–22 mU/ml 30–250 mU/ml	6–18 u/l 5–22 μ/l 30–250 u/l
Parathyroid hormone	<10 μl equiv/ml	<10 ml equiv/l
Prolactin	2–15 ng/ml	0.08/6.0 nmol/l
Renin activity	Supine: 1.1 ± 0.8 ng/ml/h Upright: 1.9 ± 1.7 ng/ml/h Supine: 2.7 ± 1.8 ng/ml/h Upright: 6.6 ± 2.5 ng/ml/h Diuretics: 10.0 ± 3.7 ng/ml/h	0.9 ± 0.6 (nmol/l)h 1.5 ± 1.3 (nmol/l)h 2.1 ± 1.4 (nmol/l)h 5.1 ± 1.9 (nmol/l)h 7.7 ± 2.9 (nmol/l)h

THYROID HORMONES

	REFERENCE RANGE	
DETERMINATION	Conventional	SI
Thyroid-stimulating-hormone (TSH)	0.5–3.5 μU/ml	0.5–3.5 mU/l
Thyroxine-binding globulin capacity	15–25 μg T/100 ml	193–322 nmol/l
Total triiodothyronine by radioimmunoassay (T_3)	70–190 ng/100 ml	1.08–2.92 nmol/l
Total thyroxine by RIA (T_4)	4–12 μg/100 ml	52–154 nmol/l
T_4 resin uptake	25–35%	0.25–0.35
Free thyroxine index (FT_4I)	1–4 ng/100 ml	12.8–51.2 pmol/l

HEMATOLOGIC VALUES

	REFERENCE RANGE	
DETERMINATION	**Conventional**	*SI*
Coagulation factors:		
Factor I (fibrinogen)	0.15–0.35 g/100 ml	4.0–10.0 μmol/l
Factor II (prothrombin)	60–140%	0.60–1.40
Factor V (accelerator globulin)	60–140%	0.60–1.40
Factor VII-X (proconvertin-Stuart)	70–130%	0.70–1.30
Factor X (Stuart factor)	70–130%	0.70–1.30
Factor VIII (antihemophilic globulin)	50–200%	0.50–2.0
Factor IX (plasma thromboplastin cofactor)	60–140%	0.60–1.40
Factor XI (plasma thromboplastin antecedent)	60–140%	0.60–1.40
Factor XII (Hageman factor)	60–140%	0.60–1.40
Coagulation screening tests:		
Bleeding time (Simplate)	3–9 min	180–540 seconds
Prothrombin time	Less than 2 second deviation from control	Less than 2-second deviation from control
Partial thromboplastin time (activated)	35–37 seconds	25–37 seconds
Whole-blood clot lysis	No clot lysis in 24 hours	0/d
Fibrinolytic studies:		
Euglobulin lysis	No lysis in 2 hours	0 (in 2 h)
Fibrinogen split products	Negative reaction at greater than 1 : 4 dilution	0 (at >1 : 4 dilution)
Thrombin time	control ±5 s	control ±5 s
"Complete" blood count:		
Hematocrit	Male: 45–52%	Male: 0.42–0.52
	Female: 37–48%	Female: 0.37–0.48
Hemoglobin	Male: 13–18 g/100 ml	Male: 8.1–11.2 mmol/l
	Female: 12–16 g/100 ml	Female: 7.4–9.9 mmol/l
Leukocyte count	4300–10,800/mm³	4.3–10.8 × 10⁹/l
Erythrocyte count	4.2–5.9 million/mm³	4.2–5.9 × 10¹²/l
Mean corpuscular volume (MCV)	80–94 μm³	80–94 f l
Mean corpuscular hemoglobin (MCH)	27–32 pg	1.7–2.0 fmol

HEMATOLOGIC VALUES *(Continued)*

DETERMINATION	REFERENCE RANGE	
	Conventional	**SI**
Mean corpuscular hemoglobin concentration (MCHC)	32–36%	19–22.8 mmol/l
Erythrocyte sedimentation rate	Male: 1–13 mm/h	Male: 1–13 mm/h
	Female: 1–20 mm/h	Female: 1–20 mm/h
Erythrocyte enzymes:		
Glucose-6-phosphate dehydrogenase	5–15 U/g Hb	5–15 U/g
Pyruvate kinase	13–17 U/g Hb	13–17 U/g
Ferritin (serum)	0–20 ng/ml	0–20 µg/l
Iron deficiency	Greater than 400 ng/l	>400 µ/l
Iron excess		
Folic acid		
Normal	Greater than 1.9 ng/ml	>4.3 mmol/l
Borderline	1.0–1.9 ng/ml	2.3–4.3 mmol/l
Haptoglobin	100–300 mg/100 ml	1.0–3.0 g/l
Hemoglobin studies:		
Electrophoresis for abnormal hemoglobin		
Electrophoresis for A₂ hemoglobin	1.5–3.5%	0.015–0.035
Hemoglobin F (fetal hemoglobin)	Less than 2%	>0.02
Hemoglobin, met- and sulf-	0	0
Serum hemoglobin	2–3 mg/100 ml	1.2–1.9 µ mol/l
Thermolabile hemoglobin	0	0
Lupus anticoagulant	0	0
L.E. (lupus erythematosus) preparation:		
Method I	0	0
Method II	0	0
Leukocyte alkaline phosphatase:		
Quantitative method	15–40 mg of phosphorus liberated/h/10¹⁰ cells	15–40 mg/h
Qualitative method	Males: 33–188U	33–188 U
	Females (off contraceptive pill) 30–160 U	30–160 U
Muramidase	Serum, 3–7 µg/ml	3–7 mg/l
	Urine, 0–2 µg/ml	0–2 mg/l
Osmotic fragility of erythrocytes	Increased if hemolysis occurs in over 0.5% NaCl; decreased if hemolysis is incomplete in 0.3% NaCl	

(Continued)

HEMATOLOGIC VALUES *(Continued)*

	REFERENCE RANGE	
DETERMINATION	**Conventional**	*SI*
Peroxide hemolysis	Less than 10%	>0.10
Platelet count	150,000–350,000/mm³	$150–350 \times 10^9/l$
Platelet function tests:		
Clot retraction	50–100%/2 h	0.50–1.00/2 h
Platelet aggregation	Full response to ADP, epinephrine and collagen	1.0
Platelet factor 3	33–57 s	33–57 s
Reticulocyte count	0.5–1.5% red cells	0.005–.015
Vitamin B_{12}	90–280 pg/ml (borderline: 70–90)	66–207 pmol/l (borderline: 52–66)

CEREBROSPINAL FLUID VALUES

	REFERENCE RANGE	
DETERMINATION	**Conventional**	*SI*
Bilirubin	0	0 μmol/l
Cell count	0–5 mononuclear cells	
Chloride	120–130 meq/l	
Colloidal gold	00000000000001222111	same
Albumin	Mean: 29.5 mg/100 ml ±2 SD: 11–48 mg/100 ml	0.295 g/l ±2 SD: 0.11–0.48
IgG	Mean: 4.3 mg/100 ml ±2 SD: 0–8.6 mg/100 ml	0.043 g/l ±2 SD: 0–0.086
Glucose	50–75 mg/100 ml	2.8–4.2 mmol/l
Pressure (initial)	70–180 mm of water	70–180 arb. u.
Protein:		
Lumbar	15–45 mg/100 ml	0.15–0.45 g/l
Cisternal	15–25 mg/100 ml	0.15–0.25 g/l
Ventricular	5–15 mg/100 ml	0.05–0.15 g/l

MISCELLANEOUS VALUES

	REFERENCE RANGE	
DETERMINATION	**Conventional**	**SI**
Ascorbic acid load test	0.2–2.0 mg/h in control sample	0.3–3.2 nmol/s
	24–49 mg/h after loading	38–77 nmol/s
Autoantibodies		
Thyroid colloid and microsomal antigens	Absent	
Stomach parietal cells	Absent	
Smooth muscle	Absent	
Kidney mitochondria	Absent	
Rabbit renal collecting ducts	Absent	
Cytoplasma of ova, theca cells, testicular interstitial cells	Absent	
Skeletal muscle	Absent	
Adrenal gland	Absent	
Carcinoembryonic antigen (CEA)	0–2.5 ng/ml, 97% healthy nonsmokers	0–2.5 μg/l, 97% healthy nonsmokers
Chylous fluid		
Cryoprecipitable proteins	0	0 arb. unit
Digitoxin	17 ± 6 ng/ml	22 ± 7.8 nmol/l
Digoxin	1.2 ± 0.4 ng/ml	1.54 ± 0.5 nmol/l
	1.5 ± 0.4 ng/ml	1.92 ± 0.5 nmol/l
Duodenal drainage:		
pH	5.5–7.5	5.5–7.5
Amylase	Over 1200 U/total sample	>1.2 arb. u
Trypain	Values from 35 to 160% "normal"	0.35–1.60
Viscosity	3 min or less	180 s or less
Gastric Analysis For hydrochloric acid	Basal:	0.6 ± 0.5
	Females 2.0 ± 1.8 meq/h	
	Males 3.0 ± 2.0 meq/h	0.8 ± 0.6 μmol/s
	Maximal: (after histalog or gastrin)	4.4 ± 1.4 μmol/s
	Females 16 ± 5 meq/h	
	Males 23 ± 5 meq/h	6.4 ± 1.4 μmol/s
Gastrin-1	0–200 pg/ml	0–95 pmol/l
Immunologic tests:		
Alpha-fetoglobulin	Abnormal if present	
Alpha 1-Antitrypsin	200–400 mg/100 ml	2.0–4.0 g/l
Antinuclear antibodies	Positive if detected with serum diluted 1 : 10	
Anti-DNA antibodies	Less than 15 units/ml	
Bence Jones protein	Abnormal if present	
Complement, total hemolytic	150–250 U/ml	

(Continued)

MISCELLANEOUS VALUES *(Continued)*

DETERMINATION	REFERENCE RANGE	
	Conventional	*SI*
C3	Range 55–120 mg/100 ml	0.55–1.2 g/l
C4	Range 20–50 mg/100 ml	0.2–0.5 g/l
Immunoglobulins:		
IgG	1140 mg/100 ml Range 540–1663	11.4 g/l 5.5–16.6 g/l
IgA	214 mg/100 ml Range 66–344	2.14 g/l 0.66–3.44 g/l
IgM	168 mg/100 ml Range 39–290	1.68 g/l 0.39–2.9 g/l
Viscosity	1.4–1.8	
Iontophoresis	Children: 0–40 meq sodium/liter, Adult: 0–60 meq sodium/l	0–40 mmol/l 0–60 mmol/l

□ **Appendix H
FUNDAMENTALS OF RESPIRATORY
GAS EXCHANGE: THE DEFINITIONS
AND DERIVATIONS**

Allen C. Norton

GAS CONCENTRATIONS AND PARTIAL PRESSURES

Gas concentrations are expressed as a *percentage* or a *fraction*. In gas mixtures, the percentage of each component reflects the ratio of that component to the total volume:

Gas percentage = (volume of component/total volume) × 100

Example: If you fill an anesthesia bag with 200 ml of O_2 and 800 ml of N_2 the composition in the bag will be:

Total volume = volume O_2 + volume N_2
= 200 ml + 800 ml = 1000 ml
Percent O_2 = (vol O_2/total volume) × 100
= (200 ml/1000 ml) × 100 = 20% O_2
Percent N_2 = (800 ml/1000 ml) × 100 = 80% N_2

Respiratory gas measurements are frequently expressed as fractions (F) rather than as percentages:

Gas fraction = gas percentage/100

("Divided by 100" is what percentage means. Examples: 80% = .80, .0050 = 5.0%, .2093 = 20.93, etc.)

The *amount* of one gas in a mixture equals the product of the concentration of that gas and the total volume.

From the example above:

Amount = volume × concentration
1000 ml × 20% O_2 = 200 ml O_2

Note: This basic mixing equation is used in many respiratory and metabolic calculations such as the Haldane transformation, calculation of oxygen uptake, determination of dead space and residual volume.

PARTIAL PRESSURE (GAS TENSION)

The concept of partial pressure of gases in mixture is not as intuitively obvious as that of concentration, although it is related to the concentration.

Each gas in a mixture exerts a pressure.

The total pressure is the sum of the partial pressures.

The partial pressure of each gas is proportional to its concentration in the mixture.

Gas pressures and partial pressures are expressed in mm Hg or torr (1 torr is 1 mm Hg). At sea level the total atmospheric pressure is 760 mm Hg.

Partial pressure = concentration × total pressure

The partial pressure of O_2 at sea level is:

.2093 × 760 mm Hg = 159.1 mm Hg

You can also calculate the concentration of a gas from its partial pressure and the total pressure.

Concentration = partial pressure/total pressure

Example: The partial pressure of O_2 in alveolar air is about 100 mm Hg. Find the concentration for a patient in Tucson, Arizona, which has a barometric pressure of 700 mm Hg:

100 mm Hg/700 mm Hg = .1429 = 14.29% O_2

Note: These partial pressure equations apply only for gases in gaseous mixtures. The situation is different when gases are dissolved in liquids. The behavior of gases in liquids is discussed in a subsequent section.

WATER VAPOR AND THE RESPIRATORY GASES

As the respiratory gases pass over the moist tissues in the air passages, they become saturated with water vapor at 37°C. This adds 47 mm Hg of water partial pressure to the gases. The result is:

The total pressure remains the same.

The new mixture includes 47 mm Hg water vapor

The remaining (dry) gases are diluted in the new mixture.

Example of an expired air sample:

$$16\% \ O_2 + 4\% \ CO_2 + 80\% \ N_2 = 100\%$$

At barometric pressure $(P_B) = 750$

$$PO_2 = .1600 \times 750 = 120 \text{ mm Hg}$$
$$PCO_2 = .0400 \times 750 = 30 \text{ mm Hg}$$
$$PN_2 = .8000 \times 750 = 600 \text{ mm Hg}$$

When humidified:

$$P(\text{dry gases}) + P(H_2O) = 750 \text{ mm Hg}$$
$$P(\text{dry gases}) = 750 \text{ mm Hg} - 47 \text{ mm Hg} = 703 \text{ mm Hg}$$
$$PO_2 = .1600 \times 703 = 112 \text{ mm Hg}$$
$$PCO_2 = .0400 \times 703 = 28 \text{ mm Hg}$$
$$PN_2 = .8000 \times 703 = 563 \text{ mm Hg}$$

The opposite occurs when a gas sample is dried, for example a humidified sample:

$$15\% \ O_2, \ 5\% \ CO_2, \text{ balance } N_2$$
$$(\text{alveolar gas}) \quad PH_2O = 27 \text{ mm Hg and } P_B = 745 \text{ mm Hg}$$
$$.15 \times (745 - 27) = 109 \text{ mm Hg } O_2$$

and

$$.05 \times (745 - 27) = 36 \text{ mm Hg } CO_2$$

after drying:

$$.15 \times 745 = 112 \text{ mm Hg } O_2 \text{ and } .05 \times 745 = 37 \text{ mm Hg } CO_2$$

THE GAS LAWS

The *kinetic molecular theory* of gases states that gas molecules behave like point sources of mass that fill the volume in which they are contained. They exert a pressure on their container which increases as more molecules strike the surface; the pressure also increases as the molecules strike the surface moving faster.

Boyles' law states that when you compress a fixed amount of gas, volume decreases and pressure increases; when you expand the gas, volume increases and pressure decreases. The equation is:

$$P \times V = \text{Constant}$$

or for different conditions:

$$P_1 \times V_1 = P_2 \times V_2$$

With any three conditions known, you can solve for the other. *Example:* A 3-liter syringe is stoppered and compressed to 2.75 liters; initial pressure was 760 mm Hg, what is the final pressure?

$$760 \text{ mm Hg} \times 3 \text{ liters} = ? \times 2.75 \text{ liters}$$
$$(3 \text{ liters} \times 760 \text{ mm Hg})/2.75 \text{ liters} = 829 \text{ mm Hg}$$

Charles' law states that a fixed amount of gas sample will increase in volume as the temperature increases and decrease as the temperature decreases. Temperature is expressed in degrees absolute (273 + °'s C).

$$V/T = \text{Constant}$$

or for different conditions:

$$V_1/T_1 = V_2/T_2$$

Example: A sample of gas occupies 6 liters at 37°C. What volume does it occupy at 0°C?

$$6 \text{ liters}/(273 + 37) = ?/273$$
$$(6 \text{ liters} \times 273)/(273 + 37) = 5.3 \text{ liters}$$

The *general gas law* combines Boyles' and Charles' laws, stating that the volume of a gas is inversely proportional to the pressure and directly proportional to the absolute temperature.

$$(P \times V)/T = \text{Constant}$$

or for different conditions:

$$(P_1 \times V_1)/T_1 = (P_2 \times V_2)/T_2$$

Solving for V_2:

$$V_2 = V_1 \times (P_1/P_2) \times (T_2/T_1)$$

BTPS volume corrections use this general gas law formula to correct the volume of gas measured to the volume that same gas occupied in the body.

ATPS   Ambient Temperature (as measured), T_1
      Ambient Pressure (barometric pressure, P_B) P_1
      Saturated (at measured temp) PH_2O

BTPS   Body Temperature $T_2 = 37°C$
      Ambient Pressure (P_B) P_2
      Saturated (at 37°C) $PH_2O = 47$ mm Hg

Since the pressure of the dry gases influences the volume, subtract the water vapor pressure from ambient pressure for the two different conditions. Thus:

$$P_1 = P_B - PH_2O \text{ (at } T_1)$$
$$P_2 = P_B - 47 \text{ mm Hg}$$

Thus,

$$V_{BTPS} = V_{ATPS} \times \frac{P_B - PH_2O}{P_B - 47} \times \frac{273 + 37°}{273 + T_1}$$

STPD volume corrections are used to correct metabolic gas flows (VO_2 and VCO_2) to standard temperature and pressure.

STPD   Standard Temperature, $T_2 = 0°C$
        Standard Pressure, $P_2 = 760$
        Dry ($PH_2O = 0$)

from ATPS measurements:

$$V_{STPD} = V_{ATPS} \times \underset{\substack{\text{Boyles'} \\ \text{law}}}{\frac{P_B - PH_2O}{760}} \times \underset{\substack{\text{Charles'} \\ \text{law}}}{\frac{273}{273 + T_1}}$$

from BTPS conditions (as previously calculated):

$$V_{STPD} = V_{BTPS} \times \frac{P_B - 47}{760} \times \frac{273}{273 + 37}$$

combining constants:

$$V_{STPD} = V_{BTPS} \times \frac{P_B - 47}{863}$$

MINUTE VOLUME

The calculations above apply to static volumes. When a volume of gas is collected over a period of time, you express this as the average flow over that time to give the minute volume, as follows:

$$\dot{V}_E = \text{(Volume accumulated/Time [sec])} \times 60$$

Note: A dot is placed over the V to indicate flow, the first derivative of volume in minute volume and metabolic gas flows, thus:

$$\dot{V}_E, \dot{V}O_2, \dot{V}CO_2.$$

Since the respiratory pattern is cyclic (inspiration followed by expiration, etc.), the time of volume collection should be for a fixed number of breath cycles, not for a fixed interval (say one minute). This is achieved by starting and ending the timed interval at corresponding points in the respiratory cycle (onset of inspiration for example).

Note: By convention minute volume ($\dot{V}_E$) and alveolar ventilation ($\dot{V}_A$) are reported under BTPS conditions with a temperature of 37° even if the patient has a different body temperature. Metabolic gas exchange ($\dot{V}O_2$ and $\dot{V}CO_2$) is always reported for STPD conditions. STPD conditions allow determination of the chemical amount of gas, since one mole (gram molecular weight) of a gas occupies 22.4 liters at standard temperature (0°C) and pressure (760 mm Hg).

TIDAL VOLUME AND RESPIRATORY RATE

With the count of the number of breaths (num) during the interval $\dot{V}_E$ is measured, tidal volume (V_T) and respiratory rate (f_r) are calculated as follows:

$$V_T = \dot{V}_E/num \quad \text{(the average volume in each breath)}$$
$$f_r = num/time\ (sec) \times 60 \quad \text{(Breaths/min)}$$

The V_E is obviously the product of tidal volume and rate:

$$\dot{V}_E = V_T \times f_r$$

METABOLIC CALCULATIONS

The basic metabolic calculations are O_2 uptake ($\dot{V}O_2$) and CO_2 production ($\dot{V}CO_2$). The O_2 consumed is the difference between the O_2 inhaled and the O_2 exhaled:

$$\dot{V}O_2 = \text{amount } O_2 \text{ in} - \text{amount } O_2 \text{ out}$$

The *amount of gas* in a sample is the product of the concentration of that gas in the sample and the volume in the sample. We use the qualifiers I and E to indicate inspired and expired volumes (V) and concentrations (F).

$$\dot{V}O_2 = (F_IO_2 \times \dot{V}_I) \times (F_EO_2 \times \dot{V}_E)$$

constant | measured | measured
unknown

It may not be immediately obvious that the inspired volume does not equal the expired volume. When the RQ is 1.00, exactly the same number of CO_2 molecules is used as the O_2 molecules used. But for all other conditions, the CO_2 exhaled will be less (usually) or more (occasionally) than the O_2 used. Since different amounts of gas occupy different volumes, it is necessary either to measure or to calculate the $\dot{V}_I$. Failure to do this results in errors of about 6% at the extremes of the RQ range.

Solving for $\dot{V}_I$ uses the *Haldane transformation,* which is based on the fact that N_2 is neither produced nor consumed in human respiration. The consequence of this is that there is the same amount of N_2 in the inspired and expired air. We express that:

$$F_IN_2 \times \dot{V}_I = F_EN_2 \times \dot{V}_E$$

Solving for $\dot{V}_I$:

$$\dot{V}_I = \dot{V}_E \times (F_EN_2/F_IN_2)$$

Substituting into the equation for $\dot{V}O_2$, we obtain:

$$\dot{V}O_2 = [\dot{V}_E \times (F_EN_2/F_IN_2) \times F_IO_2] - (F_EO_2 \times \dot{V}_E)$$

Factoring $\dot{V}_E$ gives:

$$\dot{V}O_2 = \dot{V}_E \times \{[(F_EN_2/F_IN_2) \times F_IO_2] - (F_EO_2)\}$$

Note: For systems that measure the inspired volume, the Haldane transformation is solved for $\dot{V}_E$. Notice also that although it is mathematically correct to measure the N_2 in the exhaled air, most systems measure CO_2 since this is needed for subsequent measurement of $\dot{V}CO_2$ and RQ.

When CO_2 is measured, the N_2 may be determined from *Dalton's law,* which states that the total pressure of a gas mixture is equal to the sum of the partial pressures of its components. For a respiratory gas sample:

$$P_{tot} = PO_2 + PCO_2 + PN_2$$

Dividing both sides by P_B expresses this as fractions:

$$1 = FO_2 + FCO_2 + FN_2$$

Solving for N_2:

$$FN_2 = 1 - FO_2 - FCO_2$$

This expression may be used both for F_IN_2 and F_EN_2. Substituting into the $\dot{V}O_2$ equation gives:

$$\dot{V}O_2 = \dot{V}_E \times \left\{\left[\frac{(1 - F_EO_2 - F_ECO_2)}{(1 - F_IO_2 - F_ICO_2)} \times F_IO_2\right] - F_EO_2\right\}$$

This is the basic calculation formula for $\dot{V}O_2$. The formula includes true O_2, which is occasionally reported in itself. It is important as an intermediate step in the determination of oxygen uptake which includes the terms for all of the gas concentration measurements but does not include volume. The true O_2 is the difference in O_2 between the inspired and expired air corrected for differences between the inspired and expired volumes but without the need to measure the volume. It is a useful term in error analysis of metabolic measurements:

$$TO_2 = \left[\frac{(1 - F_EO_2 - F_ECO_2)}{(1 - F_IO_2 - F_ICO_2)} \times F_IO_2 \right] - F_EO_2$$

NORMALIZING OXYGEN UPTAKE TO BODY WEIGHT

Oxygen uptake is often expressed as oxygen consumed (in ml) per unit body weight (in kg).

$$\dot{V}O_2/kg = \dot{V}O_2/(\text{Body weight})$$

An alternative is to express oxygen uptake as METS; METS are multiples of the resting $\dot{V}O_2$. In this application one MET is taken as 3.5 ml oxygen uptake per kilogram of body weight:

$$\text{METS} = \dot{V}O_2/(\text{Body weight} \times 3.5)$$

CARBON DIOXIDE PRODUCTION ($\dot{V}CO_2$)

Since inspired air contains little CO_2, it is not necessary to use the Haldane transformation to account for the difference between the inspired and the expired volume. Slightly increased accuracy is obtained, especially in some applications, by measuring the F_ICO_2 and F_ECO_2 and using the difference in the calculation of VCO_2:

$$\dot{V}CO_2 = \dot{V}_{E(STPD)} \times (F_ECO_2 - F_ICO_2)$$

RESPIRATORY EXCHANGE RATIO (R)

The *respiratory exchange ratio* is the ratio of CO_2 produced divided by the O_2 consumed:

$$R = \frac{\dot{V}CO_2}{\dot{V}O_2}$$

We have seen above that VO_2 can be expressed as the product of true O_2 and the STPD minute ventilation. Since both $\dot{V}O_2$ and VCO_2 include the term for STPD ventilation, the ratio R can be written as:

$$R = \frac{F_ECO_2 - F_ICO_2}{\text{true } O_2}$$

As above the calculation of true O_2 is:

$$TO_2 = \left[\frac{(1 - F_EO_2 - F_ECO_2)}{(1 - F_IO_2 - F_ICO_2)} \times F_IO_2 \right] - F_EO_2$$

This convenient calculation uses only gas measurements and does not require volume measurements. It also shows that the accuracy or error of R is independent of the accuracy or error of measuring volume.

During some steady state conditions the respiratory exchange ratio (R) is the same as the respiratory quotient (RQ). The RQ is the result of cellular metabolism (again the ratio of CO_2 produced to O_2 used).

THE VENTILATORY EQUIVALENTS

The ventilatory equivalents, the indicators of gas exchange efficiency, tell how much ventilation is required to transfer one liter of O_2 or CO_2. They are simply the ratio of ventilation to gas exchange.

For O_2:

$$O_2V_E = \dot{V}_E/\dot{V}O_2 \quad \text{(Units: liters/liter)}$$

For CO_2:

$$CO_2V_E = \dot{V}_E/\dot{V}CO_2$$

Note: In this ratio V_E is expressed in liters/min BTPS while VO_2 and VCO_2 are expressed in liters/min STPD.

As an indication of efficiency of gas exchange, often only the O_2V_E is reported. The CO_2V_E is used together with the O_2V_E in determination of the respiratory anaerobic threshold.

OXYGEN PULSE

The *oxygen pulse* is the amount of oxygen ejected with each beat of the heart; the calculation uses the heart rate (f_c):

$$O_2 - pulse = \dot{V}O_2/f_c$$

DEAD SPACE

Conceptually, dead space (V_D) is the volume of the inspired tidal volume that does not participate in gas exchange. The basic measurement, however, gives the ratio of dead space to tidal volume (V_D/V_T) which is in fact a ratio of two different gas concentrations. The derivation of the calculation of V_D/V_T uses the *basic mixing equation* for calculation of the amount of a gas, in this case CO_2 in the exhaled air. For the derivation, you use alveolar gas (see below for discussion of physiological and anatomic dead space).

For *the basic equality* we note that the amount of CO_2 in the exhaled alveolar gas ($F_ACO_2 \times V_T$) is the same as the amount of

CO_2 in the expired air in which the alveolar gas is mixed with the dead space gas ($F_ECO_2 \times V_T$), thus:

$$F_ACO_2 \times V_A = F_ECO_2 \times V_T$$

The dead space is the difference between the alveolar volume and the tidal volume:

$$V_D = V_T - V_A$$

Solving for alveolar volume,

$$V_A = V_T - V_D$$

Substituting for V_A in the above:

$$F_ACO_2 \times (V_T - V_D) = F_ECO_2 \times V_T$$
$$(F_ACO_2 \times V_T) - (F_ACO_2 \times V_D) = F_ECO_2 \times V_T$$

Solving for V_D:

$$F_ACO_2 \times V_D = (F_ACO_2 \times V_T) - (F_ECO_2 \times V_T)$$
$$V_D = [(F_ACO_2 \times V_T) - (F_ECO_2 \times V_T)]/F_ACO_2$$

Dividing by V_T:

$$V_D/V_T = \frac{F_ACO_2 - F_ECO_2}{F_ACO_2} = 1 - \frac{F_ECO_2}{F_ACO_2} \quad \text{(anatomic)}$$

When alveolar CO_2 is used for this measurement, the dead space defined is called the *anatomic dead space.*

By using arterial CO_2 pressure ($PaCO_2$), a similar derivation gives the physiological dead space:

$$V_D/V_T = 1 - \frac{PaCO_2}{P_B \times F_ECO_2} \quad \text{(physiological)}$$

Note: The calculation of anatomic dead space uses the ratio of gas fractions while the physiological dead space calculation converts the mixed venous F_ECO_2 to a partial pressure to match the same units (mm Hg) as the $PaCO_2$ given from a blood gas analyzer.

The volume of the dead space may be calculated from the V_D/V_T and the V_T:

$$V_D = (V_D/V_T) \times V_T$$

When measurements are made with some breathing apparatus, such as a non-rebreathing valve, the dead space indicated will include that of the subject and the apparatus dead space (ADS). The patient's dead space is determined by subtraction:

$$V_D = V_DTOT - ADS$$

The latter may be divided by tidal volume for the ratio.

ALVEOLAR SPACE

The *alveolar space* is the difference between tidal volume and the dead space:

$$V_A = V_T - V_D$$

ALVEOLAR VENTILATION

The *alveolar ventilation* that passes through the active parts of the lungs is the difference between the total ventilation (minute volume) and the dead space ventilation:

$$\dot{V}_A = \dot{V}_E - \dot{V}_D$$

The dead space ventilation is the product of the dead space and the respiratory rate:

$$\dot{V}_A = \dot{V}_E - (f_r \times V_D)$$

GASES IN LIQUIDS

The discussion of gas concentrations and partial pressures above applies to gaseous mixtures. As the respiratory gases dissolve in liquids, an equilibrium is established between the fluid and the gas mixture. The partial pressure in liquid phase is the same as the partial pressure in the gas phase. However, while the amount of gas can be determined from the partial and total pressures in the gas phase, the amount of gas in the liquid phase depends upon the solubility of the particular gas in the particular liquid. Unlike most solids, the solubility of most gases decreases as the temperature of the liquid increases. For any one temperature the amount of gas dissolved in a liquid increases with increasing partial pressures. Oxygen is quite insoluble in aqueous solutions. At body temperature (37°C), the solubility of oxygen in blood is only about .03 ml O_2 per dl of liquid per mm Hg of PO_2. You can express the content of oxygen in water (w) as:

$$CwO_2 = PO_2 \times .03 \quad \text{(Units: ml } O_2/\text{dl liquid)}$$

Very little oxygen is carried as physically dissolved in the blood.

HEMOGLOBIN

In addition to being soluble in the blood, oxygen combines chemically with the hemoglobin in the red blood cells to carry large amounts of O_2. Each gram of hemoglobin (Hb), when fully saturated, can carry 1.34 ml of oxygen. The normal Hb concentration in human adults is 12 to 15 g/dl.

OXYGEN SATURATION

As hemoglobin is exposed to increasing partial pressures of oxygen its saturation increases. The relation between partial pressure (P_xO_2) and saturation (S_xO_2) is known as the *oxygen dissociation curve*. The dissociation curve is not linear. Above $P—CO_2$s of about 90 mm Hg the hemoglobin is almost completely saturated; the S_xO_2 shows little or no increase with large increases in the P_xO_2. Below P_xO_2s of about 75 mm Hg the saturation drops rapidly with decreasing P_x. The temperature and pH of the blood result in slight shifts of the dissociation curve.

OXYGEN CONTENT

The amount of oxygen carried by the hemoglobin in the blood (Ca or CvO_2) is a function of the hemoglobin concentration and its saturation:

$$C_xO_2 = 1.34 \times Hb \text{ (g/dl)} \times S_xO_2 \text{ (\%)}$$

The total amount of oxygen in the blood also includes the small amount of physically dissolved O_2:

$$C_xO_2 = (1.34 \times Hb \times S_xO_2) + (P_xO_2 \times .03) \qquad \text{(Units: ml } O_2/\text{dl)}$$

THE FICK EQUATION

The Fick equation expresses the amount of blood passing through the pulmonary circulation, the exchange of the respiratory gases $(\dot{V}O_2$ and $\dot{V}CO_2)$, and the change in the content of the respiratory gases in the blood during gas exchange. This is an important relationship because the amount of blood passing through the pulmonary circulation is the same as that passing through the systemic circulation cardiac output.

The Fick equation states that the amount of oxygen absorbed in the lungs is equal to the amount of blood passing through the lungs (Q) times the difference between the content of oxygen in the venous blood arriving in the lungs (CvO_2) and that in the arterial blood leaving the lungs (CaO_2):

$$\dot{V}O_2 = \dot{Q} \times (CaO_2 - CvO_2)$$

This is an interesting concept: oxygen uptake can be calculated from measurement of $\dot{Q}$ and C_xO_2 in arterial and venous blood. In many situations VO_2 can be measured but cardiac output is more difficult to determine. The Fick equation, however, can be solved for Q and thus cardiac output can be calculated from measurement of VO_2 and the difference in content between the arterial and mixed venous blood.

$$\dot{Q} = \frac{\dot{V}O_2}{CaO_2 - CvO_2}$$

NONINVASIVE CARDIAC OUTPUT

The Fick equation may be used in the same way to estimate cardiac output from CO_2 rather than O_2. Like oxygen, carbon dioxide uses the naturally occurring respiratory gas rather than a foreign tracer gas. The advantage of using CO_2 is that the arterial and venous CO_2 contents may be estimated from noninvasive maneuvers which do not require drawing blood samples through indwelling catheters. The basic principle is similar to the O_2 Fick equation. It states that the amount of blood flowing through the pulmonary circulation ($\dot{Q}$) is equal to the CO_2 produced ($\dot{V}CO_2$) divided by the difference in CO_2 content between the arterial and venous blood ($CvCO_2 - CaCO_2$):

$$\dot{Q} = \frac{\dot{V}CO_2}{(CvCO_2 - CaCO_2)}$$

$\dot{V}CO_2$ is measured directly.

End tidal CO_2 ($P_{ET}CO_2$) is used to estimate $PaCO_2$. There is an empirical correction from $P_{ET}CO_2$ to $PaCO_2$ which in some cases improves the estimate of pulmonary blood flow:

$$PaCO_2 = 5.5 + (0.9 \times P_{ET}CO_2) - (2.1 \times V_T) \quad \text{(Optional)}$$

$CaCO_2$ is calculated as a function of $PaCO_2$. This is an expression of the CO_2 dissociation curve. The equation as expressed by McHardy is:

$$CaCO_2 = 11.02 \times (PaCO_2)^{.396} \quad \text{(Units: ml } CO_2\text{/dl)}$$

Mixed venous CO_2 is estimated from a rebreathe procedure during which the gas mixture in the lungs and rebreathing bag ($P_{bag}CO_2$) is brought into equilibrium with the $PvCO_2$ in blood arriving in the pulmonary artery. Here too there is an empirical correction, sometimes called the "downstream" correction, which is used to improve the estimate of pulmonary blood flow:

$$PvCO_2 = P_{bag}CO_2 - (0.24 \, P_{bag}CO_2 - 11)$$

Mixed venous CO_2 content ($CvCO_2$) is calculated from the CO_2 dissociation curve:

$$CvCO_2 = 11.02 \times (PvCO_2)^{.396} \quad \text{(Units: ml } CO_2\text{/dl)}$$

The difference between venous and arterial CO_2 content can be calculated combining the corrected P_xCO_2s:

$$(CvCO_2 - CaCO_2) = 11.02 [(PvCO_2)^{.396} - (PaCO_2)^{.396}]$$

This calculation describes differences along the CO_2 dissociation curve for nominal hemoglobin concentrations (Hb = 15 gm/dl) and oxygen saturation ($SaO_2 > 95\%$). When Hb or SaO_2 differ, the following correction is used:

$$(CvCO_2 - CaCO_2)_{corrected} = (CvCO_2 - CaCO_2)$$
$$- .015 \times (PvCO_2 - PaCO_2) \times (15 - Hb)$$
(Hb correction)
$$- .064 \times (95 - SaO_2)$$ (SaO_2 correction)

Thus we see the elements of the equation:

measured directly
|
$$\dot{Q} = \frac{\dot{V}CO_2}{(CvCO_2 - CaCO_2)}\text{—corrected for Hb and } SaO_2$$

from end tidal corrected to arterial

from rebreathe corrected for "downstream"

Note: When end tidal samples and samples from the rebreathing are measured undried, but remote from the mouth, the samples which initially included a water vapor pressure of 47 mm Hg will have less water vapor. The amount of water vapor remaining in the sample is related to the lowest temperature to which the gas is exposed before it is analyzed. Some water vapor will "rain out" before the gas is analyzed. The loss of water from the sample enriches the remain gases. Thus while the partial pressure of CO_2 at body temperature should have been 47 mm Hg, a higher valve will be measured. This affects the conversion of these gases from fractions to partial pressures as follows:

$$PCO_2 = FCO_2 \times (P_B - P_{orig}H_2O + P_{lost}H_2O)$$

Measurements by myself and others of the change in the partial pressures in partially humidified gases indicate the loss of about 18 mm Hg water vapor sampling through unheated sample lines of about 1.5 m at an ambient temperature of about 22°C. Thus:

$$PCO_2 = FCO_2 \times (Pb - 47 \text{ mm Hg} + 18 \text{ mm Hg})$$
$$= FCO_2 \times (Pb - 29 \text{ mm Hg})$$

CALCULATIONS USING CARDIAC OUTPUT

Both cardiac output and energy expenditure are often indexed to *body surface area* (BSA). BSA is calculated from height (Ht) and weight (Wt) using the formula of DuBois (height is in cm and weight in kg):

$$BSA = 71.84 \times Wt^{.425} \times Ht^{.725} \times 10^{-4} \quad \text{(Units: square meters)}$$

The *cardiac index* (CI) is the cardiac output Q indexed to body surface:

$$CI = \dot{Q}/BSA \quad \text{(Units: liters/min/m}^2\text{)}$$

Stroke volume (SV) is calculated from $\dot{Q}$ and heart rate f_c:

$$SV = \dot{Q}/f_c \quad \text{(Unit: ml/beat)}$$

Stroke volume index (SVI) is the stroke volume indexed to body surface area:

$$SVI = SV/BSA \quad \text{(Units: ml/beat/m}^2\text{)}$$

METABOLIC CALCULATIONS

The Harris-Benedict equations predict resting energy expenditure (REE in Cal/day) on the basis of height (cm), weight (kg), age (yr), and sex.

For males:

$$REE = (13.7 \times Wt) + (5.0 \times Ht) - (6.8 \times Age) + 66$$

For females:

$$REE = (9.6 \times Wt) + (1.7 \times Ht) - (4.7 \times Age) + 655$$

These predictive equations represent averages. They do not account for individual differences or the effects of drugs or disease.

Measured energy expenditure can be determined by indirect calorimetry. One liter of oxygen produces about 5 Cal of energy. There are slight differences in the energy produced by the different substrates which are accounted for by the differences in the $\dot{V}O_2$ and $\dot{V}CO_2$ in the *Weir equation*:

$$\text{Energy (Cal)} = (3.80 \times \dot{V}O_2) + (1.20 \times \dot{V}CO_2)$$

When $\dot{V}O_2$ and $\dot{V}CO_2$ are in liters/min, energy expenditure is in Cal/min.

A frequently used variant of the Weir equation is:

$$\text{Energy expenditure} = (3.94 \times \dot{V}O_2) + (1.11 \times \dot{V}CO_2)$$

Experimentation with substituting values for $\dot{V}O_2$ and $\dot{V}CO_2$ shows there is very little difference in the energy expenditure calculated by the different versions of the Weir equation.

The resting energy expenditure (REE) is usually expressed in Cal/day. Liters/min are converted to liters/day as follows:

$$\text{liters/day} = \text{liters/min} \times 60 \text{ min/hr} \times 24\text{-hr/day} = 1440$$

The daily resting energy expenditure of a patient measured at rest may be expressed:

$$\text{REE (Cal/day)} = 1440 \times [(3.796 \times \dot{V}O_2) \times (1.214 \times \dot{V}CO_2)]$$

WHAT ABOUT URINARY NITROGEN?

Nitrogen excretion indicates the amount of protein oxidized. Most (but not all) nitrogen is eliminated in the urine. A nitrogen balance study requires measurement of all nitrogen lost: urine, stool, wounds, etc. (It is a difficult, tedious, and often inexact procedure.) Ignoring nitrogen loss in indirect calorimetry results in very very small errors in calculation of energy expenditure estimates. For substrate partitioning, you must measure urinary nitrogen.

SUBSTRATE PARTITIONING

For substrate partitioning, collect a 24-hour urine sample and analyze for grams nitrogen per day. Determine the total or average $\dot{V}O_2$ and $\dot{V}CO_2$ for the same 24-hour period.

When urinary nitrogen is measured (UN) and analyzed for a 24-hour period and combined with the average gas exchange for that same period, there are calculations which indicate the substrates utilized.

The first step is to calculate the $\dot{V}O_2$ and $\dot{V}CO_2$ per day by multiplying the liters per minute by 1440.

Next, empirical constants are used to determine the amounts of substrates (carbohydrates [CHO], lipids [FAT] and protein [PRO]) oxidized:

$$\text{grams CHO oxidized} = (4.115 \times \dot{V}O_2) - (2.909 \times \dot{V}CO_2) - (2.56 \times \text{UN})$$
$$\text{FAT oxidized} = (1.689 \times \dot{V}O_2) + (1.689 \times \dot{V}CO_2) - (1.94 \times \text{UN})$$
$$\text{PRO oxidized} = (6.25 \times \text{UN})$$

When the RQ > 1.00, there is a net fat synthesis. Different equations must be used:

$$
\begin{aligned}
\text{grams CHO oxidized} &= (1.393 \times \dot{V}CO_2) - \\
&\quad (0.187 \times \dot{V}O_2) - \\
&\quad (2.539 \times UN) \\
\text{FAT synthesized} &= (1.689 \times \dot{V}CO_2) - \\
&\quad (1.689 \times \dot{V}CO_2) - \\
&\quad (1.943 \times UN) \\
\text{PRO oxidized} &= (6.25 \times UN)
\end{aligned}
$$

The grams of CHO converted to FAT equal 2.83 multiplied by the grams FAT synthesized.

The amount of calories produced by each substrate is the product of the grams oxidized and its efficiency (more empirical constants):

$$
\begin{aligned}
\text{Cal/day CHO} &= 4.18 \times \text{CHO g/day} \\
\text{Cal/day FAT} &= 9.46 \times \text{FAT g/day} \quad \text{(for FAT oxidation)} \\
&= -1.089 \times \text{FAT g/day} \quad \text{(for FAT synthesis)} \\
\text{Cal/day PRO} &= 4.32 \times \text{PRO g/day}
\end{aligned}
$$

When substrates are calculated individually, the total energy expenditure may be calculated from the sum of the substrates:

$$
\text{Total Cal} = \text{Cal CHO} + \text{Cal FAT} + \text{Cal PRO}
$$

Note: Only slight differences between the above calculation and the Weir equation occur when UN is not reported.

NONPROTEIN RQ

The *nonprotein RQ* reflects the relative amounts of carbohydrates (RQ = 1.00) and lipids (RQ = .70) being oxidized. It is determined by the ratio of the $\dot{V}CO_2$ not contributing to protein oxidation divided by the $\dot{V}O_2$ not contributing to protein metabolism.

First calculate the $\dot{V}O_2$ and $\dot{V}CO_2$ accounted for by protein oxidation:

$$
\begin{aligned}
\text{UN g/day} \times 5.92 &= \dot{V}O_2 \quad \text{(for protein oxidation)} \\
\text{UN g/day} \times 4.75 &= \dot{V}CO_2 \quad \text{(for protein oxidation)}
\end{aligned}
$$

Then calculate the nonprotein (NP) gas exchanges:

$$
\begin{aligned}
\dot{V}O_2 NP &= \dot{V}O_2 TOT - \dot{V}O_2 PRO \\
\dot{V}CO_2 NP &= \dot{V}CO_2 TOT - \dot{V}CO_2 PRO
\end{aligned}
$$

Finally, the ratio is calculated:

$$
RQ_{NP} = \frac{\dot{V}CO_2 NP}{\dot{V}O_2 NP}
$$

DILUTION OF EXPIRED GASES

Measurement of gas exchange requires accurate measurement of both the expired volume and the expired gas concentrations. Since gas exchange is the product of the volume of and difference in gas concentrations, when either is measured incorrectly the product will be in error. Similarly when there is a violation of the integrity of either the volume (loss of sample or addition of extraneous sample) or gas concentration (removal of some component or dilution with some other gas), the product—gas exchange—will be in error. The maintenance of sample integrity is extremely important. Gas leaks and contaminations can not be tolerated.

There is, however, a situation in which the expired air sample may be diluted before it is measured. This is *when the expired air is diluted with inspired air*. In this situation the volume increases, the exhaled gases are diluted, but the product (gas exchange) remains constant.

This is easily seen for $\dot{V}CO_2$:

$$\text{For: } \dot{V}_E = 6000 \text{ ml/min } F_ECO_2 = .0400$$
$$\dot{V}CO_2 = 6000 \times .0400 = 240 \text{ ml/min}$$

When diluted by 6000 ml of inspired air:

$$\dot{V}_E = 6000 + 6000 = 12000 \text{ ml/min}$$
$$F_ECO_2 = [(6000 \times .0400) + (6000 \times 0)]/(6000 + 6000)$$
$$= .0200$$

Then: $\dot{V}CO_2 = 12000 \times .0200 = 240 \text{ ml/min}$

The insensitivity to dilution with inspired air may be less obvious for VO_2 and RQ.

Expanding the example above, the patient's basic gas exchange is as follows:

$$\dot{V}_E = 6000 \text{ ml/min} \qquad F_IO_2 = .2093 \qquad F_ICO_2 = .0003$$
$$F_EO_2 = .1600 \qquad F_ECO_2 = .0400$$
$$\dot{V}O_2 = \left\{ \left[\frac{(1 - .1600 - .0400)}{(1 - .2093 - .0003)} \times .2993 \right] - .1600 \right\} \times 6000$$
$$= 311 \text{ ml/min}$$
$$\dot{V}CO_2 = [(.0400 - .0003) \times 6000 = 240 \text{ ml/min}$$
$$RQ = 240/311 = .77$$

If in a canopy or IMV ventilator with blow-by the patient's exhaled air is diluted with 27,000 ml/min room air flowing past the patient, the expired gases are diluted as follows:

$$F_ECO_2 = [(.0400 \times 6000) + (.0003 \times 27000)]/(6000 + 27000)$$
$$= .0075$$
$$F_EO_2 = [(.1600 \times 6000) + (.2093 \times 27000)]/(6000 + 27000)$$
$$= .2003$$

Solving for gas exchange with the diluted exhaled gases and expanded volumes gives:

$$\dot{V}O_2 = \left\{ \left[\frac{(1 - .2003 - .0075)}{(1 - .2093 - .0003)} \times .2093 \right] - .2003 \right\} \times 33000$$
$$= 312 \text{ ml/min}$$

$\dot{V}CO_2 = [(.0075 - .0003) \times 33000 = 238 \text{ ml/min}$
$RQ = 238/312 = .76$

The calculations shown use the numbers rounded as indicated; the slight differences are solely the result of rounding errors.

index

The letter *f* after a page number indicates a figure; *t* following a page number indicates tabular material.